ADVANCE PRAISE FOR

Balance Is Power

"Training balance is essential for enhancing the quality of human movement. Jim Klopman is a pioneer in the integration of balance training for improving not only quality of movement but quality of life."

— DANA SANTAS CSCS, E-RYT, PRO SPORTS
MOBILITY COACH AND CNN YOGA EXPERT

"Jim's groundbreaking balance equipment and balance training protocols have been the single most important component of human performance training that I have seen in the last two decades."

— JAKE SWEENEY, OWNER,
JAKE'S HOUSE OF IRON

"The next best thing to training in person with the balance master himself is picking up this book and using it as a bible, not only for better balance, but better living. Practicing what Jim preaches, even without a commitment of much time or effort, has tuned my body and mind in ways that no other discipline has. I don't know anyone over the age of ten who doesn't need this book."

—SUSAN ADES STONE, AWARD-
WINNING JOURNALIST

"When I started using the protocol with my clients, I was amazed at how quickly their balance improved. [I worked with] a 16-year-old competitive rifle shooter. Prior to utilizing the SlackBow, his average score hovered around 156 out of 200. After 12 sessions with the SlackBow, and no other changes in his training protocol, his score had increased to an astounding 186. He recently qualified for the Junior Olympics."

—JOHN JARMAN, OWNER & HEAD COACH,
SUMMIT STRENGTH & CONDITIONING

"I would rather lose my sense of hearing than my sense of balance. Fortunately, with Jim's experience anyone can improve their sense of balance which impacts all areas of well being, and is the defining trait of all athletics and sports."

— TYLER CROWLEY

"Everyone: young, old, fit, frail, elite athletes or weekend warriors should read this book. Klopman is right; by using his tools to develop your balance you can improve performance in any sport, maintain general health and well being, recover better from injuries, and prevent falls in the elderly. So no more excuses, buy this book!"

— CELESTE RAFFIN, MD

BALANCE IS POWER

Balance is
POWER

Improve Your Body's Balance *to* Perform Better, Live Longer, *and* Look Younger

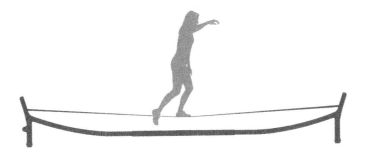

Jim Klopman

with Janet Miller

BALANCE IS POWER

*Improve Your Body's Balance to Perform
Better, Live Longer, and Look Younger*

ISBN   978-1-61961-458-1   *Paperback*
         978-1-61961-459-8   *Ebook*

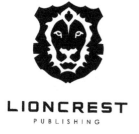

To you, who believed before all others:
Katie Fike and Betsy Sanders; my life force and daughters
Janet Miller; my partner in everything and muse
Susan Ades Stone; a brilliant and generous advisor

Contents

———

Introduction

===

Would a lifelong golfer believe me if I told him that at age sixty-seven he would be shooting the best score of his life after a few brief sessions of basically standing on one leg? How about a middle-aged skier, an Olympic-style marksman, or a basketball player? Would they believe me if I told them they would ski their fastest, shoot their finest, or improve their vertical leap by at least 10 percent without so much as practicing their sport, lifting weights, or enduring even a single movement drill?

Would a Division 1 football strength coach believe that his team's injury rate would drop by working tiny muscles his players can't even see? Or would someone with post-concussion syndrome believe she could be relieved of chronic and debilitating neurological symptoms by working on the micro-muscles that keep her upright?

Would architects, digital product designers, eyeglass makers, or athletic shoe manufacturers believe me if I told them their creations were compromising the body's major neural information system, leading to declines in productivity and cognitive performance while increasing the number of falls that land people in emergency rooms or, even worse, in their graves?

Would you believe me?

Five years ago, I would not have believed any of this myself. However, in my determination to become an even better athlete as I age, I discovered the holy grail of fitness that changed me both physically and cognitively. Along the way, I had the privilege of sharing my growing knowledge with hundreds of athletes—weekend warriors and pros—and watching their lives transformed. I designed equipment and protocols that helped people improve performance both physically and mentally. So with this book, I aim to convince you—and the world—that all of the above is not only true but also easily achievable if you just understand and believe in the power of balance.

Marketers may say, "Where's your research?" Fitness trainers may say, "C'mon, nothing can be that easy." But consider Charles Darwin. He came back from the Galapagos Islands to report that animals develop their adaptive traits based on their environment, not based on divine design. The scientific community demanded proof, and he explained that his was but a theory backed by observations and only time could prove him right.

So, I say, don't wait for the scientists. My buddy Dave Asprey, pioneer "biohacker" and author of the *New York Times* best-selling *The Bulletproof Diet* says we each need to be our own scientist. Researchers want sample sizes of hundreds, but your sample size is one and it is you, because, really, what do you have to risk by improving your balance? Do the work in this book and watch the results. The proof won't be bigger muscles but improved productivity, improved athletic performance, better sleep, better mood, and I'm convinced, longer life. I'm not guaranteeing you'll never fall again. But if you do, your body will instinctively know how to recover your step to avoid serious injury. And all of these benefits will come with a minimum of cost, time, and effort.

Every once in a while, there is a universal shift in the understanding of how to achieve optimal health. No doubt we are living longer. And, yes, habits like good diet, exercise, and meditation are important, but something has been missing from the instruction manual for tuning the human machine to enable tip-top performance throughout a good, long life. And that is balance training.

If the body and the brain are our hardware, balance is our operating system. It's time for a reboot. And I'm here to be your guide.

Part One

WHY BALANCE
MATTERS

Balance: Our Sixth and Most Important Sense

═══

YOUR JOURNEY

Here is a stark fact: In the United States, the number of deaths from falls has nearly doubled from 2000 to 2013. And this is despite the boom in fitness training, stricter building codes that eliminate fall hazards, and improvements in accessibility. At the same time, the United States has been in the throes of a revolution in health care, struggling with how to pay for it, who gets it, and how to keep people out of the emergency room (ER), where the cost of care is more expensive. According to the US Centers for Disease Control and Prevention, in 2011 half of all visits made by people age forty-five and over were for falls. Many of those falls could have been prevented if people had spent the little time it takes to keep their balance system healthy.

Here is my theory: The modern lifestyle is dealing a serious blow to the human balance system. In primitive times, our balance was constantly challenged by the uneven ground and varied terrain that we traveled every day. Now, we move in a world designed to protect us from falls—smooth, even sidewalks, exceptionally flat floors, and perfectly proportional stairs. A crack in the pavement is cause for complaints and yellow tape to warn us away from the hazard. Perfectly aligned living and work spaces are not the only causes of our balance loss. You can add electronic digital screens, universally poor shoe design, archaic fitness methods, and even eyeglasses.

Restoring our natural maximal balance has nothing to do with building new muscles or developing new skills. It is not about, as the saying goes, teaching an old dog new tricks. In fact, it is difficult to describe how rapidly the body resets its sense of balance without invoking the word *magic*. The fact is, with minimal effort, the body's balance system has a way of simply rebooting itself.

Bulking up is entirely unnecessary in acquiring good balance. Look no further than the world of professional sports, and you'll see that the best athletes are seldom shaped like a weightlifter. A big-muscle physique does not equate in any way whatsoever with good balance. Often, an athlete who has great balance will resemble that of the iconic Roman sculpture: long, smooth muscles.

Balance training goes well beyond the making of the super successful athlete, as those who participate in the exercises achieve results in cognitive and emotional performance in unnatural settings, such as the office or the classroom. The depleting effects on the body of those rectilinear indoor environments, where much of modern life is spent, can be warded off to a large extent by reengaging the balance system.

Improved balance will quickly make you a better athlete, but it can also, without hyperbole, literally be the difference between life and death for any of us planning on living to a healthy old age. How is it possible to prevent falling and suffering injury? The best way is to begin improving balance sooner rather than later. Therefore, now is the best time. That said, it is never too late to begin balance training.

My aim in writing this book is that the reader will take a journey into new developments in the field of advanced balance training, giving it a solid go, to see what personal discoveries are to be made. Clients testify that it is "mind-blowing" how quickly advances take place not only in terms of balance skills, but also in the overall positive effect it has on one's whole life.

Here is our guarantee: When you launch into the program, you will begin a rewarding lifelong discipline to achieve and maintain your optimal balance. And in so doing, you will find a harmonious balance in *everything* you do.

BALANCE: OUR SIXTH AND MOST IMPORTANT SENSE

Balance—why is this one sense, which is so indispensable to survival and key to all athletic success, so widely misunderstood?

The sense of balance is comprehended innately, much like our olfactory sense. No one "teaches" us that roses smell pleasant or that bovine flatulence doesn't. We know these things instinctively. Be that as it may, our sense of smell has deteriorated over several millennia as our other senses have become more critical in organized societies.

The smell of a wolf at five hundred yards might have been the difference between life and death for a nomadic hunter, whereas for a sophisticated city dweller behind large walls and armed with projectile weapons, a stronger sense of hearing, for example, might be more crucial to survival, as important information began being delivered audibly with the use of words, rather than olfactorily by the use of varying scents.

In the same way, this modern, civilized lifestyle has put us out of touch with our sense of balance. That invaluable skill that once allowed our primitive ancestors to stealthily stalk prey or gather herbs from hard-to-reach locations has diminished over time. Little balance is required to move from desk to break room to restroom and back to desk.

As I stated before, the result of this atrophying of balance skills is that more than half of the people over the age of forty-five who go to the ER are there because they have fallen down. And to be clear, that is just the ER visits; many falls do not require immediate emergency medical attention, yet an injury can still happen.

It is common for people to assume, "That's just other people. That won't happen to me because I have good balance." That line of thinking, however, often lulls people into a fall sense of confidence. There is a mistaken belief that good balance is like some kind of genetic trait that some people have and others lack, and that this trait is permanent and requires no maintenance.

As a matter of fact, athletic, physically fit people suffer these falls. Having never so much as stumbled, they possess an overconfidence or a blind spot that someone with a history of falling or a known lack of balance is wary of.

There are three excuses I get when I ask my clients how their fall happened.

1. *"I wasn't paying attention."* Of course they weren't paying attention. No one pays attention when they are walking unless they have bad balance. Walking is a mindless activity in which we do everything but pay attention.

2. *"There was a problem with my shoes."* Sure there was. That's why there are so many class action lawsuits against Nike and Adidas for faulty footwear design, and why the federal government instituted the National Shoe Safety Board, which goes door to door conducting random shoe inspections. (I am being sarcastic of course.)

3. *"I have not had any problems with falling before."* Translation: "I had no idea that my balance had degenerated."

These explanations illustrate a lack of understanding about the sense of balance. There is a tendency to think that good balance means not teetering while standing or walking. However, there is a vast difference between the balance required to stand straight and the native, movement-based balance hidden within us. I say "hidden" because this inborn sense of balance has been obscured by the forces of modern life, which shield us from honing the sense, resulting in its deterioration—that is, until a fall happens.

The sense of balance is evident in sports, and there is a clear connection between it and athletic prowess. That said, the value of athletic balance is misunderstood, and attempts to identify it become trite. For instance:

"He runs with great agility and balance."

"She swings with great balance."

"He moves with grace and balance."

These generic statements demonstrate the vague connection between balance and exceptional athletic performance. It is universally seen but has no clear definition. Agility and coordination are directly related to an athlete's balance skills, but no one seems to understand why. That's why I began studying that relationship.

What I've learned is that the best athletes in a sport are the ones who also have the best balance. That's not a coincidence. My unique view is that balance is part of the autonomic nervous system, functioning involuntarily without conscious control. The balance system regulates all body movements, with the primary purpose of preventing falls. One feature of this regulatory system is that a body's attempted movements are allowed or disallowed based on the person's skill level with regard to balance. In other words, this system works to prevent the body from executing maneuvers above its balance pay grade.

For example, suppose a professional football receiver is asked to run a ten-yard "out" pattern. He is expected to sprint ten yards down the field, deceiving the defender into thinking he is going to continue in that direction, but instead, he must turn on a dime, so to speak, and break hard—ninety degrees—toward the sideline, where the ball will be arriving simultaneously. That's the idea in theory anyway.

In practice, that receiver is either going to decelerate into his break or is going to take a wide, arcing turn toward the sideline. Why is this the case? It's because each individual body has a level of balance that determines how quickly and how sharply that route can be run. The receivers with better balance skills will execute that sprint-and-cut with greater velocity and a straighter angle. Receivers with lesser balance will run slower and turn wider or they will stumble and fall, and probably roll like a top-heavy SUV taking a sharp turn at high speed. The autonomic protective balance system will prevent his falling by slowing him down. The receiver may have the muscles and skills to turn faster. His balance system will not allow him to go faster.

To improve one's speed and agility, one merely needs to work on one's balance skills. The training is far easier, ridiculously quicker, and the results are astronomically more significant than any other. In this book, I address some of the components of balancing for every athletic movement.

There is a misconception that has been spread that performance enhancement requires hard work. *No pain, no gain.* There is something almost comforting about believing that athletic gains are the fruit of physically exhausting toil for which there is no shortcut. There seems to be something fair about that. But that's not how the body works. The relationship between effort and results is not a one-to-one ratio. It is actually possible to get far more out of the work you put in if you put in the *right* work.

I know this sounds too good to be true. On the surface, it sounds a little like magic. One of my skiing clients, after just a couple of hours of training, was so incredulous of his rapid improvement—he was skiing comfortably much faster—that he accused me of hypnotizing him.

A skier has an internally created speed limit that subconsciously calculates the measurement of slope difficulty combined with velocity. That speed limit is based on his or her balance skill level. As the skier approaches her internal speed limit, the autonomic nervous system kicks in. "Maybe I should slow down," she thinks. When she exceeds her internally set speed limit, real fear sets in, and the body's autonomic system of balance involuntarily reacts to slow her down.

Human balance is an extremely complex multimodal neural system. Establishing balance is of primary concern to the body. Before it will commence with any other activity, the body will first seek to balance itself. So controlling is this system that like the skier whose body will slow itself beyond a certain speed, it will also limit how fast a person is capable of walking. People with bad balance are incapable of even walking at the same speed as those who have good balance. Past a certain age, walking speed is a sign of longevity. The faster you are able to walk, the longer you will live.

In fact, the consequences are even more far reaching. Imagine a baseball player at the plate. A pitch is thrown. The batter's idea is to hit the ball squarely. This ability to make solid contact with the ball is based primarily on the sense of balance.

Balance is very complicated compared to the other senses. The sense of vision, for instance, takes information that the eyes have gathered and sends it to the brain, where it is converted into images. The sense of hearing does the same thing with sounds, using the ears. Balance, on the other hand, gathers information from a variety of sources. The primary source is the vestibular organ, which, although located inside the ear, is not used for hearing. The vestibular is considered the "balance organ," the one organ dedicated to balance. Even so, there are many other sources of information the entire balance system relies on: proprioception; mechanoreception, especially on the bottom of the foot; and the eyes.

But beyond these conventionally known sources of information, other inputs also seem to aid in balance. The tongue, one of the most nerve-dense parts of the body, may be one such source. My observations are that the tongue takes on a unique position while balancing, and maybe nerves are being stimulated. Exactly how and why that's the case is the subject of further research.

When I observe my clients, I see that the palms of the hands also appear to play a role in balance. Like the tongue, the palms are rich in nerve endings. In fact, there are more nerve connections to the palms than to any other part of the body. My clients' palms consistently move to a common position while performing balance challenges.

What is remarkable is that all of these systems work symbiotically in unison to create nanosecond-by-nanosecond adjustments to our daily movements. Even if you think you are standing still, these interconnected systems are constantly working hard. Even if it can't be observed, movement is taking place. It is impossible to stand perfectly still despite how motionless the royal guard at Buckingham Palace appears. The fact is, thousands of micro-movements per second are necessary just to keep the body vertical and stationary.

The body is naturally in a perpetual state of imbalance. Myriad forces are at work to knock us over, but the balance system is making fast-as-light calculations and small adjustments to correct for the imbalances. What we refer to as "balance" is, ironically, thousands of micro-movements that when combined give the appearance of stillness.

To illustrate that, consider the movement of electrons, which whir around the atom's nucleus at such high speed that the individual electron cannot be seen, only the elliptical path it travels. So, too, our many micro-movements cannot be detected, only the result: a seemingly motionless standing body.

The balance system separates us from the rest of the mammal kingdom. Apes and other primates will sometimes stand on two feet, as will bears. Most four-legged animals have the ability to stand on two legs. Humans are the only mammals specifically designed to stand on two legs, or for that matter, one leg.

This system requires a massive amount of neural bandwidth and muscle activation, which explains why merely standing up can be so tiring, thus making the act of leaning against something so appealing. In doing so, the hardworking balance system is disengaged. This rare ability to balance is essential in making human beings the successful species that we are. Why, then, do we pay so little attention to our sense of balance, considering it only after injury occurs?

Like any need that modernity has eliminated, the issue seemed resolved. The precivilization need for a strong sense of balance, like a strong sense of smell, that our ancestors survived on had become supplanted by a lifestyle that was made more ergonomically comfortable by new technologies and less balance-reliant methods of labor.

People who live closer to nature in rural areas use their balance to a greater extent. The old expression holds true: *Use it or lose it.* The sense of balance, like any skill, atrophies with disuse.

Anthropologist Kathryn Linn Geurts, author of *Culture and the Senses: Bodily Ways of Knowing in an African Community*, has researched indigenous tribes to determine which bodily senses are most important in the raising of their children. While researching the Anglo Ewe-speaking people of Ghana, Geurts asked them to rank the traditionally understood five senses—hearing, vision, smell, taste, and touch—in order of importance. The Anglo Ewe expressed surprise that she had left off her list the most important sense of all: balance.

Lying down is the only activity you can do without your sense of balance. Without balance, the human body is incapable of sitting, standing, or accomplishing any type of athletic movement. It is the one sense that exerts the most control over the human experience.

BALANCE BEYOND SPORTS

My research into the sense of balance has not been merely to improve the performance of skiers and football players. I have been skiing since I was four; I lettered in five sports in high school. Even apart from that, I was a physically reckless young man and have had more than my share of concussions.

A recent brain scan revealed that I had the same type of

damage as that of an ex-NFL player who has had multiple concussions. The area in my brain with the most damage is my cerebellum, the part of the brain that is supposed to operate the balance system. (See photo in chapter 16.)

Despite this damage, I contend that there are maybe a handful of people my age with my balance skills. I had unwittingly found my way into the study of balance as a means of repairing my damaged neural control system, figuring that balance training would help with the kinds of problems that I and some former professional football players face. Even before my brain scan, I'd had the sense that improving my balance would help rewire my brain for the better.

My instincts were correct. And the implications turned out to be even broader than I could imagine. My methods of balance training have had remarkable success helping others trapped in post-concussion syndrome break free of their concussion symptoms and get back to enjoying an active life.

KLOPMAN BALANCE INDEX

I have studied every possible balance test available and to be honest, none of them measured what I was looking for. For the purposes of what I will be explaining in the pages that follow, I will spare the reader a review of those shortcomings.

To better explain what balance is—and can be—I have created an index to measure this misunderstood ability. The Klopman Balance Index (KBI) is a 0–100 scale. The major markers are not hard-and-fast precision points, as it is currently a theoretical model. Major points on the scale are as follows:

- *0 – No balance system; lying down is all that can be done*
- *20 – The point at which a cane or walking stick is needed*
- *60 – Weekend warrior-level balance*
- *75 – College/pro athlete*
- *85+ – The very best athletes (Wayne Gretzky, Steph Curry, Jordan Spieth)*
- *95+ – Cirque du Soleil and circus balance performers*

One of my reasons for creating the scale is because the spectrum of balance is actually much wider than what is currently understood for athletes. For example, a young skier with post-concussion syndrome was referred to me. His mother asked why he needed to do my training even after a physical therapist had cleared him. I suggested he come in for a KBI test. His balance was fair, and it was easy to understand why he was cleared by his physical therapist to continue skiing.

He measured about 50–55 on the KBI scale, which is a mediocre measurement for a skier. However, this young man competed in slopestyle competition, performing flips, rail slides, and backward actions. To compete at that level, one needs to have a minimum score of 70. I explained that to him and his mother, and he trained with me. When he finished, he was above 80 on the scale. Not only did he recover from his concussion symptoms, but he also became a better skier.

The human body's potential with regard to improving balance is far greater than is commonly conceived. My clients are shocked by the balance challenges they are able to execute on their first day of training. They are doing techniques they assumed to be not only impossible but also dangerous within an hour.

CHAPTER 2

Why Are We So Off-Balance?

"That's a first-world problem," my son-in-law, Jim, tells me after I complain about my cell phone service. He wants me to know that in terms of third world, less-developed countries, my complaint is trite, and that as a first worlder, I should be thankful to be living in a wealthy and prosperous country such as the United States.

Setting aside poor use of outdated terms, such as "third world," let's acknowledge that even in developed nations, there are serious problems that need to be addressed—obesity, attention deficit hyperactivity disorder (ADHD), autism, and Alzheimer's disease immediately come to mind. And if I might add another issue to that ever-growing list, I would include the deterioration of balance, which has yet to be fully understood by the scientific community, although it is now being studied as a serious topic as the facts below illustrate:

- The National Institutes of Health is funding a $30 million study on balance.
- There are more than 40,000 neuroscientists worldwide, many of whom currently study body movement and balance.

The epidemic of fall-related injuries and deaths is, as my son-in-law likes to say, a first-world problem. In my view, the loss of balance in developed countries can be linked to architectural design. In a world of perfectly flat floors, sidewalks, and stairs, there is not much, if anything, to challenge our system of balance, which becomes disengaged due to disuse. Generally, the only impediments along our smooth, flat surfaces are the occasional cracked sidewalk, pothole, or low curb—which, by the way, is one of the leading causes of falls for those over sixty-five.

Additionally, we own products that, while intended to make our lives better or easier, actually harm our balance systems by diminishing its use: for example, shoes, eyeglasses, smartphones, TVs, computers, tablets, and more.

ARCHITECTURE

The human balance system has suffered decay due to the effects of the modern office and school environments. Simply going about daily life inside an office or classroom is a factor in the atrophy of balance.

Consider what it's like to be outside, walking in a forest on a winding trail. The natural environment is made up of uneven shapes, such as leaves, trees, and rocks. There are no square or rectangular shapes to be found in nature and certainly nothing that resembles our perfectly smooth, geometrically perfect modern habitat. These randomly shaped objects in nature are composed of only fractal surfaces.

So contrast that forest with the office with its cubicles and linear hallways, square and rectangular rooms, and other "unnatural" designs. Even the grid outside of the office, with its straight roads (in most cities anyway), train tracks, sidewalks, buildings, and other structures, is a rectilinear world.

With its unpredictability in footing and variances in spatial relationships, the forest and other wilderness areas require attention to balance. The exactitude of a staircase, however, requires only measuring the distance of a single step and then repeating that motion until we are back on the flat surface of another level that requires little in the way of attention to balance.

The modern world is designed to be stumble-free lest lawsuits be filed or building codes be made more stringent. A mere raised crack in the floor of a public building or a spilled glass of water causes that area to be cordoned off until maintenance crews can fix it.

Modern spaces are built to accommodate the least balanced among us, people who require canes, walkers, and wheelchairs—people with a Klopman Balance Index (KBI) score of 20–25. I'm not for a moment suggesting that we don't create a mobile-friendly environment for the walking impaired; I'm only pointing out that this ease has degraded the sense of balance for those with adequate balance or better. The purpose of this book is to help the reader restore the loss of balance skills.

If a majority of one's life is spent in a stumble-free world, that person's balance system will degrade to a KBI of 25–35. When a balancing challenge occurs at a KBI of, say, 45, that person will stumble, maybe fall, and maybe sustain an injury.

So, if our sense of balance can atrophy because of disuse, what else is in store for someone who spends most, if not all, of his or her time in the rectilinear predictability of man-made environments?

We innately understand and feel the negative effects of hours spent inside an office. Do you ever hear anyone say, "Hey, we need to spend more time in the office"? No, of course not. What is always said is, "We need to get out of the office more. We need to get outside." It is often said, in fact, that sitting is the new smoking. We are only now beginning to understand the dangers of a sedentary low-balance-challenge life.

Retreats are popular part of corporate culture. Retreats occur in natural settings. Outdoor sports, such as golf, skiing, and hiking are common bonding activities. Another is the ropes course, which builds self-confidence, improves team cohesiveness, and creates better decision making. These things are said to occur because of the value of risk taking and the pushing-through of self-imposed limits. While those are important, there seems to be something else going on that is not altogether consciously planned.

The ropes course is a safe and aggressive balance challenge that resets the neural system. The improved self-confidence, cohesion with coworkers, and clearer thinking are directly related to the balance-challenge aspect of the ropes course. We naturally feel and perform better after our balance system has been fully activated.

Humans seek out balance challenges to reset this all-encompassing neural system, whether we realize that's one of the reasons we are doing it or not. Cycling, skiing, motorcycling, riding roller coasters, surfing, hiking, golfing, playing tennis, and many more physical activities make us feel good. The common denominator they all have is that they present challenges to our balance, and one of the reasons we enjoy these activities is because of that.

After facing the balance challenges of a sport or physical activity on a retreat or just on the weekend, the body's neural system is returned to a more natural state. When that person goes back to the office on Monday, it will be with a clear and productive mind-set. Think about it, who looks forward to Monday? Nobody. How about Friday? Everybody.

DIGITAL MYOPIA

Walls, floors, ceiling panels, fluorescent light tubes, and cubicles are not the only contributors to our depleted balance. The system also atrophies as a result of being visually glued to a smartphone, computer, tablet, or TV. Looking at these devices hurts the sense of balance because in addition to walking among rectilinear surfaces, we are now intently staring at them.

Myopia, or "nearsightedness," as we commonly refer to it, has doubled in the last fifty years. A theory among researchers of the subject is that this occurs as a result of being indoors too much. It is assumed that indoor lighting does not aid in the development of the eyes as well as sunlight does.

I'd like to offer a competing theory, which proposes that when a person spends too much time looking at something that is only about an arm's length away, his or her vision becomes atrophied beyond that distance. In other words, when someone stares at electronic screens, his or her eyes will only work effectively at that distance and will therefore require glasses for long-distance vision.

Regarding balance loss, there is a much bigger problem being caused by this myopia. Staring at and focusing on a screen causes the brain to disregard information received by the eye's peripheral vision. Balance requires broad vision and long-distance focus. Hyperfocusing on a screen disregards information from the periphery. Believe it or not, fully engaging the sense of vision really does improve balance.

I call this "peripheral vision denial," a condition in which the brain is denying the massive amount of data coming in through the peripheral vision. You see examples of this every day when people walk into each other while looking at their phone. I am six foot one. The other day, a man, about five foot seven, was stepping into an elevator as I stood in the doorway. He was looking at his phone and bumped into me. How the heck could he not see me? Easy—he had shut down that part of his brain that uses the information coming in from his peripheral vision. In his case, I hope it is not permanent. The popular photo below is a great example of peripheral vision denial.

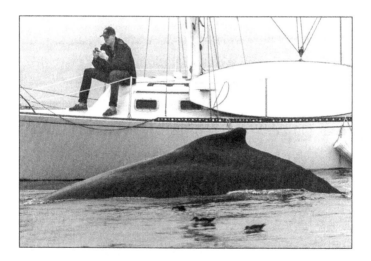

Even our electronic overlords—the computer and tech companies—instinctively know this about the soul-sucking effect of their magical electronic boxes. Apple products' screen background selections revolve around either beautiful photos of nature or fractal geometric designs. The computer companies seem to know that their rectangular boxes could be neurologically disrupting, so they compensate for that fact by employing subconsciously pleasant background images.

EYEGLASSES

The lower part of progressive or bifocal glasses is designed for up-close vision, such as reading. If, however, you focus through that part of the lens while walking, the ground is a blur. To compensate, you have to bend your head forward and down to look through the upper part of the lens. As a result, you end up using your direct vision to see the ground rather than your peripheral vision, which is a key component in accessing full balance capabilities. People wearing progressive or bifocal glasses are forced to walk head-down to see the ground through the upper part of the glasses. Ask anyone what it was like the first few days they wore their progressive lens, and they will tell you that they felt like they were losing their balance.

Ironically, we are concerned, and legitimately so, about

poor posture resulting from staring into smartphones, particularly among the younger segment of the population. However, bear in mind that older members of society who wear these glasses suffer the same problem with posture.

I ask my clients with progressive lenses or bifocals to remove their glasses. I make sure there is a safety touch-point for them nearby, and I also stay close enough to assist. They remark, of course, that they can't see very well, but when I ask them to hold their head up and look straight ahead, they are able to maintain better balance. This is because peripheral vision does not require glasses, as centrally focused vision does. Because this balance information from the peripheral vision goes directly to the subconscious, autonomous balance system, it is difficult to measure the acuity of peripheral vision.

SHOES

Just about all shoes, even top-of-the-line athletic shoes, negatively affect your balance. While that might sound counterintuitive, read on.

If you own a pair of running shoes, set one shoe on a table and look at it from the side as in the following photo. Notice how the toe box of the shoe sweeps upward. Most shoes are shaped this way.

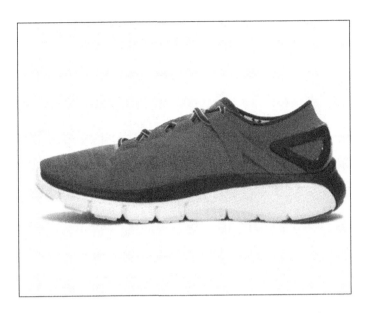

That upward sweep does not square with what we know about balance, which optimally includes one's weight forward on the forefoot and toes engaged with the ground. Walking in shoes such as these encourages the wearer to strike the ground initially with the heel.

As a thought experiment, suppose you are walking on ice, where balance is tenuous. Do you want to initially set your weight down on your forefoot or heel? If you want to stay upright, the right answer is your forefoot.

Another experiment is to just stand in your bare feet. Are you toes rolled up off the floor? Move your feet sided to side. Are you toes engaged with the floor? Why, then, are they out of contact and rolled up in your expensive shoes?

The forefoot is where most balance occurs. The big toe is the largest moving part of the foot for a reason, because it is the most important, and using it is crucial to good balance. As you look at that shoe, you'll notice that the design doesn't encourage any forefoot involvement. The most critical part of the foot is disengaged, off the ground.

Notice the rise in the heel. Most running shoes have heels, though, hidden by the thick soles, which force the wearer to stand or walk on the heels; effectively, this means being off-balance. Shoes create a situation in which the toes are off the ground, knees are locked, pelvis is rolled under, back is overarched, and heels are dug in. To get a sense of how unnatural this is, try jumping rope while bouncing off your heels. It doesn't work. There are no athletic movements that occur from your heels.

The effect is harsh. We have a hubris that assumes the foot was designed improperly, and we must remedy it with appropriate footwear. There is, to be sure, a protective purpose shoes fulfill. As a species, we wear clothes, hats, and gloves, but the heel and the turned-up fore section of the shoe are unnecessary in terms of protection.

How the heel of the shoe came into existence is unclear.

One theory is that early horseman developed it to aid in the use of stirrups but later gained popularity among the wealthy as a status symbol, demonstrating that one could afford to own horses. And for those who aspired to wealth, the heel had the effect of making one look like one owned horses. Therefore, the greater population all started wearing heels on the shoes.

There's another reason often cited for the creation of the heel. It makes one appear taller. Vanity, of course, has played a large role in the design of clothing, including footwear.

It is interesting to note that some of the greatest athletes in track and field come from countries where training barefoot is the norm. Consider, as well, that condition-specific performance shoes, such as football or baseball spikes and track shoes, do not have heels, thick soles, or turned-up toes.

In the running shoe world, the heel is referred to as "drop," which is the difference in the height between the heel and forefoot measured in millimeters. There is no consensus or valid research on how much drop is needed, although there is a great deal of passionate debate. I find it hard to believe that whole populations of extremely intelligent people wear heels on both their running shoes and street shoes, yet they are oblivious to any reason for doing so. Where is the research on why we have a raised heel? If any reader of this book knows of why we need heels on our shoes, please let me know.

When I was a kid, we all wore Chucks or similar sneakers that had no lift in the heel or turned-up forefoot.

The fact is, athletic shoes are no longer just for sports. They are fashionwear as well. The primary activities done in athletic shoes are standing, sitting, and walking, with running or training being a distant fourth.

When standing in these shoes, the main balance component of your foot—the forward third—is encouraged to be off the ground, while most of the body weight is distributed onto the heel. This forces a person into an unnatural posture and creates poor balance. This is how most people in the modern world operate for up to seventeen hours a day.

I think it is possible to gauge the athletic ability of a person by the way he or she walks. Great athletes walk with a fluid forefoot strike. However, most people walk with a strong heel strike. Some people even seem to pound the heel into the ground with a sense of authority. Interestingly enough, this heel strike only occurs on flat, artificial surfaces. On a wilderness trail uneven with rocks, stumps, and so forth, even heel strikers switch their gait to make initial impact with the forefoot.

To gauge the extent of the impact of your own heel strike, put on a pair of noise-canceling headphones or noise-isolating headphones without sound. Block all noise from without and within; in other words, don't put on music. Next, walk on a hard surface like a stone, concrete, or hardwood floor.

If you walk on your heels, you will hear a loud thump with each step. That is the shock wave created by your heel hitting the floor and reverberating all the way through your body up to your ears. Think of it in terms of a hammer hitting a block of wood. This force slams the foot into the ankle, which in turn, slams into the lower leg, and so forth, into the knee joint up to the hips. This has to cause some sort of joint damage.

Now try to walk while landing on your forefoot. You should notice a difference in that there is no sound at all. You'll also discover that it is difficult to walk on your forefoot consistently if you are not in the habit of it. There are several posture issues to deal with before it begins to feel natural, which might take months. This is one of the exercises I teach my clients.

BUILDING THE WRONG MUSCLES

The typical fitness center tends to have several dedicated rooms: a free-weight room, a weight machine room, a stretching room, a yoga room, a Pilates room, an aerobics/dancing room, and at the center of it all, a cardiovascular space with endless rows of elliptical machines, treadmills, and bikes. Where is the balance-training section of the gym?

The gym does little in the way of improving the skill of balance; instead, it offers many machines that require the user to sit down, lie down, or hold on to something. Cardio machines, for example, offer supports to hold on to, which negates the need to balance.

A seated arm curl, meanwhile, has no real connection to natural movement. Isolating individual muscles is not a part of traditional sports. Weights are mostly about building the larger muscles, but it is the smaller, stabilizer muscles that need development to generate better balance. The best athletes have better muscles, not necessarily bigger ones.

To improve balance, which improves overall athletic ability, a different type of training is necessary. It requires engaging the whole body—every muscle, every nerve—as an interconnected set of systems, just as is done naturally in athletic activity, such as sports. There is only one way to properly balance train, and it mandates the use of every part of the body.

But because we live in a world in which the need for balance has been radically reduced, why is it important to develop this sense? That is the focus of the next chapter.

INJURY AND DISEASE

It is obvious that injuries will affect balance. We like to see clients after they have finished their full physical therapy prescription. Balance training is a good follow-up to physical therapy to continue the reestablishing the small control muscles needed to prevent further injury.

We will see new clients who are having balance problems that we don't think they should have based on their general fitness and what we get from their intake form. With a little probing, we find that they had a long-ago forgotten injury. The injury left behind a muscle activation pattern that is not conducive to better balance. Oddly enough, the balance training brings back their balance and clears the compensatory muscle firing patterns from the injury.

We had a client come in one morning and said, "Watch!" He bent over and put his knuckles on the floor. I asked him what the big deal was, and he explained that he had not been able to touch his ankles ever since a blood clot was removed in his leg six months before. Every morning in the shower, he would try to touch his toes, and now he was touching his knuckles to the floor. To my surprise, this happened after two and half hours of balance training.

He had a compensatory protective muscle firing pattern from the blood clot surgery. That pattern released, and the natural correct pattern reestablished itself. It is difficult for a body to balance unless the kinetic chain is in balance.

It is clear that there is a loss of balance skills with those who have autoimmune and other types of diseases. Even though we don't see many clients in these conditions, we have seen that there is an improvement.

CHAPTER 3

The Dangers of a Weak Balance System

―――

PHYSICAL RISK

As I wrote in the introduction, fall-related injuries for people forty-five and over are a major problem. However, it is just the tip of the iceberg. The number of injuries and deaths from falls is staggering.

According to the US Department of Labor, falling is the number-one cause of industrial deaths nationwide. In 2014, falls accounted for 277,000 people being hospitalized, at a cost of $34 billion.

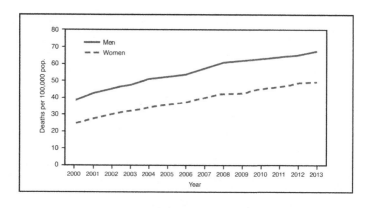

As a person ages, the outcomes of a fall can become more devastating. Look at the chart above from the Centers for Disease Control and Prevention (CDC). Age and population-adjusted deaths by falls have *increased* by 77 percent for men and 99 percent for women. During this same time, deaths from cancer have dropped nearly 20 percent. There would be outrage from all corners of society if any disease had an increase of death rates at this level.

Research compiled by the CDC underscores how important a strong sense of balance is. Roughly 25 percent of people who fall suffer moderate to severe injuries, including hip fractures, lacerations, and head trauma. In fact, most traumatic brain injuries are due to falling.

What may be most disconcerting about these statistics is that they are considered "accidents" for purposes of categorization. An accident is a freak occurrence that is unforeseeable, whereas a disease describes an existing state of deterioration.

Death caused by heart failure is termed *heart disease*. So, too, is lung failure described as a disease. However, when someone dies as a result of balance failure, it's merely an accident. To be clear, however, there exists an epidemic that can only accurately be described as a balance disease.

This epidemic has, at last, grabbed the attention of the National Institutes of Health (NIH). In 2014, the NIH, along with the Patient-Centered Outcomes Research Institute (PCORI), announced a $30-million five-year project in which they will use large-scale clinical trials to prevent falls in elderly adults, and create a "cohesive intervention" to reduce the number of falls. The project will study more than six thousand adults aged seventy-five and older.

Intervening on behalf of adults seventy-five and older with balance problems, however, is a bit like seeking an intervention for seventy-five-year-old smokers with lung cancer. To be successful in intervening, it's important to start the process much earlier. It is best to nip smoking in the bud, intervening right away to prevent lung cancer later in life. Balance, like healthy lungs, must be preserved in the same way.

A person between the ages of forty and fifty can recover the balance of youth in a very short amount of time, and can maintain it indefinitely by taking some simple steps, which I will present in this book.

PSYCHOLOGICAL IMPACTS

I have a fifty-year-old client named Jennifer who is in great shape. She doesn't play sports; instead, she gets all of her exercise from fitness classes. She says that she enjoys SlackBow Balance Training more than any other type because no matter how badly she feels emotionally before her class, she always feels better afterward. It is a recurring theme that all my clients express: balance recovery feels good physically. A properly functioning balance system is directly connected to a sense of well-being.

In 2007, Scott McCredie wrote an informative and prescient book on this subject called, *Balance: In Search of the Lost Sense*, which I highly recommend. McCredie includes in it the story of Cheryl Schiltz, a woman who lost her sense of balance after a virus destroyed her vestibular system, which, as we know, is an organ dedicated solely to balance, located in the inner ear. She could not stand or walk without holding on to something for support. In fact, she could barely sit up without falling over.

Schiltz visited the office of Dr. Paul Bach-y-Rita, who is responsible for one of the most significant discoveries ever made about the brain. He found that the brain has the ability to assign functions from its damaged areas to healthy areas, what is known as "neuroplasticity." So if a part of the brain that regulates balance is damaged, that function can, over time, be reassigned to a healthy part of the brain.

Dr. Bach-y-Rita was also an early developer of sensory prosthetics, devices designed to help people overcome one failed sense with the aid of another. For instance, he postulated that the eyes don't actually see but merely provide raw data, and that it is the brain that does the seeing. So, if a person's eyes do not work, he would find alternative methods of bringing raw image data to the "seeing" area of the brain. (For a more thorough understanding of Dr. Bach-y-Rita's work, read Norman Doidge's *The Brain That Changes Itself*, or check out the continuation of his work at the Tactile Communication and Neurorehabilitation Laboratory [TCNL] located at the University of Wisconsin.)

One of Dr. Bach-y-Rita sensory prosthetic inventions was for a failed vestibular organ. This device, which included a level attached to a helmet, would send signals to different parts of the tongue to inform the balance system which direction the body was leaning. These signals to the tongue help determine head position and movement information, and replaced the missing information from Schiltz's damaged vestibular system.

The device was designed to send information to a plate on her tongue, resulting in small pulses of electricity being delivered to different areas of the tongue. For example, if the left side of the tongue received a pulse, it meant that she was leaning left, and she could then account for that by repositioning her body. With this device, Bach-y-Rita was essentially substituting the tongue for the vestibular organ.

Within minutes of installing this device, Schiltz regained her sense of balance. What is interesting to note is that for hours after taking off the device, she retained a residual ability to balance. After each training session with the device, those residual effects lasted longer and longer. After years of suffering from imbalance, she now had a means to restore it.

Regarding the link between balance and psychological well-being, Schiltz began to experience periods of joy as the residual effects of the device lingered. In other words, while her body properly regulated its sense of balance, she felt good. However, the minute the effects wore off—and they would drop off sharply at some point—depression set in.

There are many such examples of the connection between balance and psychological health. People with Ménière's disease, a vertigo-causing condition of the inner ear, are, for example, more likely to have depression than people with any other inner-ear disease. Some people believe depression triggers Ménière's disease, but I'm of the opinion that the reverse is true: Ménière's disease causes a loss of balance, which, in turn, results in depression.

I propose that damage to the balance system could be a symptom of depression, which is a common physiological response after someone has suffered a stroke and lost the sense of balance. I am not suggesting, of course, that all depression is caused by a loss of balance, but it does appear that damaged balance leads to an onset of depression.

A walk through nature, whether in the woods, on the beach, or through the hills, improves one's sense of well-being. One reason for that, as my theory purports, is because the natural world is composed entirely of fractal surfaces, which prompt the human body to engage its sense of balance and peripheral vision. The more uneven the ground, the more our balance is challenged. And the more of a challenge, the better the sense of well-being.

Gregory Bratman, a graduate student at Stanford's Emmett Interdisciplinary Program in Environment and

Resources, studies the effects of urban living. He and his colleagues found that people who took walks in nature were more attentive and happier afterward than those who took walks in an urban environment, with its straight lines and flat, even surfaces.

Bratman and his colleagues went on to explore the possibility of a physiological effect in the brain that distinguishes between a walk in nature and an urban walk. Measuring blood flow, they saw a marked difference between the two. The study concluded that the nature walks produced a reduction in rumination, a depression-linked focus on distressing matters.

Studies indicate that walking in nature reduces stress, alleviates depression symptoms and improves overall well-being. However, is it merely the act of walking or is it the environment being traversed that matters? One study showed that runners were 50 percent happier after running outside versus running inside.

There exists a relationship between poor balance, traumatic brain injury (TBI), and depression. Half of all people with TBI suffer from anxiety as a consequence. In fact, half of people with TBI suffer from depression for a year following the injury, and nearly two-thirds still suffer from it after seven years.

Rebooting the neural system through balance training has an extraordinary effect on these negative mental states. After a series of balance challenges, the trainee's disposition changes internally, but outwardly, there are clear indications of psychological improvement visible in body language, facial expression, color, and energy.

Balance training can impact many other cognitive-related issues as well. Frank Belgau, EdD, is the developer of Balametrics, a balance program that can eliminate many, if not all, of the symptoms of dyslexia in children.

The Balametrics program also helps children with attention deficit disorder/attention deficit hyperactivity disorder (ADD/ADHD). I contend that the hyperactivity in the ADHD child is an attempt to engage and challenge an improperly functioning system of balance. Engaging and challenging that sense of balance with constant movement calms the brain.

THE WORKPLACE

Imagine for a moment the typical workplace with its cubicles, fluorescent lights, straight lines, and rectilinear geometry throughout: flat floors, ninety-degree walls, doorframes, and computer monitors. Squares and rectangles are everywhere. Even the windows, if any, are rectangular.

A worker sitting at a boxy workstation peeks out beyond a line of cubicles toward a tall filing cabinet. On top that filing cabinet, sprawling over the sides and toward the floor is a fern or a spider plant. The worker's eyes are drawn to it like a moth to flame. And why wouldn't he or she be? The living, amorphously shaped plant stands out boldly in this geometrically designed environment.

Look at the photo below. It appears to be a well-designed space. But what is the eye drawn to?

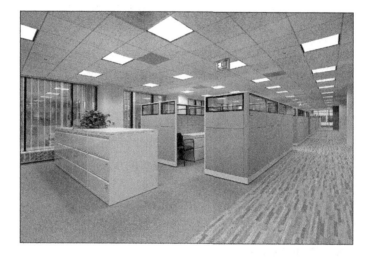

It comes as no surprise, of course, that company executives are given the perk of a window. And the larger the view, the more important the executive. What is generally not considered in this arrangement is that the window is more than just a reward; it actually energizes the worker, produces greater feelings of well-being, and clarifies thinking, ultimately generating better results.

Studies have shown that simply placing a plant on a desk can improve productivity by 15 percent. "Our research suggests that investing in landscaping the office with plants will pay off through an increase in office workers' quality of life and productivity," says lead researcher Marlon Nieuwenhuis of the Cardiff University School of Psychology.

There's a movement in the workplace in which progressive companies, such as Google, are investing in work spaces with nonrectilinear surfaces. Instead, they are focusing on providing an aesthetic that features natural curves and fractal design.

In actuality, there is a lot more that can be done besides just hanging up a plant or two. Why must an office floor be perfectly flat? Consider a slightly uneven surface, such as a cobblestone or tile floor, which pose little to no impediment in terms of causing a fall. Research, in fact, shows that elderly people are able to improve their balance by walking barefoot on cobblestone surfaces.

It is critical in discussing the redesign of the workplace to include the effects—positive or negative—on the balance system.

THE GOOD NEWS

The flood of statistics spelling out the dangers posed by a poor sense of balance—whether from disuse, poor training, or a falling accident—is vividly apparent. The good news is that I have yet to meet anyone whose balance could not be quickly improved. And part of that improvement includes the ability to function better and feel better within the rectilinear world.

CHAPTER 4

The Fix:
Rebooting the
Balance System

BALANCE IS WHAT MAKES US HUMAN

Every human movement requires balance. The human
body is incapable of walking, running, swinging an
object, standing, or even sitting without balance ability.
Just as breathing requires functioning lungs, movement
requires balance.

When we speak of a sense of balance, what is it exactly that
is being sensed? The answer remains unclear. As explained
earlier, I have defined balance as an autonomous neural
control system, and an extremely complicated one due to

the many interconnected components. With its wide array of unique input/output contributions throughout the body, it is one of the largest and most complex neural systems, extending far beyond just the vestibular organ, nerves, feet, joints, and vision. As a result, the science is still not in on many of the peculiarities of this multimodal system.

When clients begin their first session of balance work, they want to consciously control the process. This is natural because that is how we learn, say, how to hit a baseball or throw a football. There is a tendency to be very conscious in preparing to accomplish the proper movement.

High-end athletes new to the training are often the most difficult, as they know full well what their bodies are capable of, and when their bodies fail them, they naturally get frustrated, seeking to consciously override an insubordinate leg or just grab that leg and yell at it to stop shaking. What they don't understand is that the balance system essentially has its own command center, which does not relinquish control to the body it operates.

In the struggle to successfully negotiate a new balance challenge, the muscles quiver because the neural system is resetting its software. The muscles can figure out the correct firing pattern, but it takes a little time to get in sync. Just like a computer that needs to be rebooted, the body's balance system needs to reset all of its assignments and clean up its communication paths.

Martin Goulding of the Salk Institute is coauthor of a research paper titled, "Mini Brain." In it, he points out that one of the central questions in neuroscience involves the concept of the brain creating a sensory percept and turning it into an action. The balance system remains largely a mystery, partially accounting for the fact that there are currently 40,000 neuroscientists worldwide.

The metaphor I find most helpful in understanding the balance system is that of a self-correcting software system, which, when challenged, adjusts to deal with that challenge. The sense of balance fluctuates, and it does not take much to negatively affect it. I have observed clients whose balance skills had declined since previous sessions. What set them back? All it takes is having a disruptive influence. Even something as simple as having a lousy day, watching the news, or just being in a bad mood is all it takes to throw off one's sense of balance.

In such situations, I merely take that person through a series of movements that act as a neural reset program. Soon, everything starts humming again, and that person's level of balance is right back to where it used to be. It's not magic despite feelings to the contrary. It is simply a reboot of the balance software.

You might observe that you're a brilliant putter on the golf course on Wednesday, but on Friday, you can't make a four-foot putt to save your life. This inconsistency has a lot to do with balance. The same is true for other skill-type sports. If a person is performing poorly at a sport, the first question to ask is whether his or her balance system has a bug and needs a neural reset.

THE BALANCE OPERATING SYSTEM SOFTWARE

If the body and the brain are the hardware, then the balance system is the software.

Despite the fact that there are textbooks written on the subject of balance and all that it entails, I want to offer a glimpse of how complex the system is and how hard it works.

How is balance like an operating system? There are heaps of data from all over the body generated nanosecond by nanosecond and organized in a useful form to maintain balance. While the ability to walk across the street seems ordinary on its surface, there is a miraculous sensorimotor system at work to keep that body up and moving safely from point A to point B.

The vestibular organ, as mentioned, is directly involved with balance. It is comprised of three interlocking tubes containing very sensitive hair like receivers through which a fluid flows. The fluid behaves like that in a carpenter's level, moving up and down, and side to side, sending signals to the brain that the head is leaning this way or that.

Part of the genius of this design is the speed of the signal that is delivered to the brain. There are two ways to improve data delivery speed: one is to increase the rate of data throughput; the other is to place the data-generating device close in proximity to the processing source. It is clear that the human balance system is designed for fast data flow, as evidenced by the main balance organ being located right next to the brain.

The next set of data comes from the proprioceptive system. These are the sensors in muscles, joints, and fascia, which tell us the position our body is in. When you move your leg, your brain "feels" this and reacts accordingly.

Along with the proprioceptive system, there is a cartography system in the brain, which possesses a three-dimensional map of all the possible positions the body can assume. For example, if I kick my leg forward, there is a map that charts the possible positions my other leg (and torso, arms, etc.) can feasibly take in order to counterbalance my forward weight. So powerful is this mapping system that some consider it the explanation behind phantom limb syndrome—the condition in which sensation still occurs despite the loss of the appendage.

The eyes also play a crucial role in the sense of balance. Eyes are composed of rods and cones in the retina, which absorb information from the electromagnetic spectrum. The cones are concentrated in the central part of the cornea, while the rods are distributed mostly around the outside of it. The rectilinear world has created an over-reliance on the sense of direct vision, to the detriment of balance, which relies heavily on peripheral vision.

The nerve sensors on the bottom of the feet ought to be a significant component of the balance system, but because shoes counteract this input, feet do not play the central role for which they evolved. These sensors, when operating optimally, detect minute changes in the pressure they absorb, informing the body which way it is leaning.

The forefoot provides data on the shape and difficulty of the obstacle underfoot. As demonstrated on a balance-challenge course, there is a tremendous difference in balance ability between a person skilled in using the forefoot to gather information and a person who is not.

Goulding and his Salk Institute research team recently discovered that information gathered by the nerves on the bottom of the feet do not make it all the way to the brain, but are sent to brain-like cells in the spinal cord, which use this information to maintain balance. Again, like the vestibular organ, the shorter the distance that signals have to go, the faster the data processing, and thus, the sooner balance maintenance can occur.

My observation is that the hands also seem to have a role in balance, but research on the matter has yet to reveal the connection. In performing balance challenges, participants tend to position their palms in a certain way. Given the high density of nerve endings in the palm, it appears that some kind of information is being sought with those receptors. What exactly they are seeking, however, remains unclear.

The balance system is a virtual symphony of information appearing cacophonous at first; but as each individual instrument's role becomes clear, the noise then becomes melodic. There is a seemingly infinite neural network of sensors, analyzers, and stabilizers involved in maintaining balance. If anything in that network is disrupted, the whole system will sputter or even shut down entirely.

THE AUTONOMIC NERVOUS SYSTEM

The autonomic nervous system (ANS) is described in the scientific literature as a human system that is both automatic and protective. The beating heart is an example, functioning involuntarily to keep us alive despite the fact that a person can consciously speed it up or slow it down.

Other systems, not necessarily classified as an ANS, also behave similarly. The fingers, for example, feel a sting when it is really cold outside. In doing so, they are sending a message to the brain that the body needs warming. Many parts of the ANS are controllable. Take breathing—most people can hold their breath for about a minute, but people who train themselves are capable of holding their breath for seven, eight, or even nine minutes. They are able to do so by overriding powerful signals that were developed to aid in survival.

After one minute without air, the body feels like it is going to die. Panic sets in. However, it is possible to control that fear, reject that signal, and realize that death is not as imminent as it seems. This is how an ANS works. It is a protective network designed to keep the body from harm.

To date, the scientific community has not recognized the balance system as an ANS. Nevertheless, balance is a critical survival skill. When it is not functioning properly, falls ensue, resulting in injury or death. It is, indeed, a protective system. Furthermore, it is an automatic system, operating unconsciously, but unlike breathing, the balance system can't be controlled or modulated. The balance system controls your every movement. You can't turn it on or off with conscious thought like you can hold your breath.

It is impossible to hold your breath longer than your body will allow. And while that might sound like a tautology, understand that the "body" includes not just the lungs, which can be trained to hold more air, but also the brain, which can be trained to shut off the panic switch, so to speak, and allow for longer stints between inhalation and exhalation.

So, too, a person cannot move faster or turn sharper than the balance system will allow. But again, the balance system, like the breathing system, can be trained. The NFL receiver can train to maintain balance while running full speed into a ninety-degree break. A golfer can also improve his balance so that his balance system lets him swing with more power and accuracy.

THE PROCESS OF REBOOTING

Rebooting the system is not about flipping on a series of subsystems one at a time—A, B, C, D, E, and so forth. On the contrary, a reboot brings everything online simultaneously: from A straight to E. When that happens, the sense of balance is reconfigured and capable of new achievements. This rebooting process is not measured in microscopic differences but is clearly visible to the naked eye during balance training.

The key learning process powering the reboot is a type of neurological confusion, which can be very frustrating for the trainee. There are, for example, rapid movements of the leg—rapid like the stitching of a sewing machine—as signals are fired in quick succession, confusing the muscles. Those muscles appear to be arguing with each other like children discussing whose turn it is to take out the trash:

"You fire."

"No, it's your turn."

"No, I just fired. It's your turn."

For someone who has been through the training and has a highly functioning sense of balance or an elite athlete, something different altogether is going on. The same muscles are firing, but they're doing so in an organized way. They've got the timing down like a well-trained team or dance company:

"I'll fire."

"Yep, now it's my turn."

"Gotcha. Now it's my turn again."

There are telltale signs that an athlete is capable of taking his or her balance skill to another level. Interestingly, we never measure balance ability in terms of time. The fact is, when clocked, a person will become performance focused with active judgmental conscious thoughts. Like the inner game of tennis or Zen in the art of archery, balance resides beneath the conscious state of mind. Balance challenges are best met by a body that is "in the zone," so to speak, behaving autonomously out of instinct rather than volition.

When a person becomes aware of the balancing act, balance tends to be lost. Often, I will observe a person comment on the balancing challenge being performed. Inevitably, that person will fail at their challenge within three seconds of the comment. The same thing happens when I intervene to compliment a person on a balancing maneuver. Judgment is the enemy of athletic feats.

My thoughts are that once a body is at a maximum balance limit, the whole human neural network is being used to capacity; conversely, when there is any other neural load, balance is lost. Balance never occurs in isolation; we are always doing something more than balance. Once I understood this, I added in other neural challenges such as catching a beanbag while balancing. The simple acts of throwing and catching a beanbag are enough to overload the system to the point where balance is lost. The system is so sensitive that when a client is at a balance limit and I introduce, for the first time, the toss and catch, he or she loses his or her balance just from the thought of adding that one simple neural challenge.

I have not taken the Balametrics course, but they call the use of different senses at the same time "Sensory Integration." This is a good term and does explain the process. The different sensorial inputs—that is, the things we see, hear, and feel while balancing—have to be subconsciously controlled to make balance the best you can make it. Kudos to the developer, Frank Belgau. My multineural-load concept comes from his beanbag toss and catch while balancing protocols. The Balametrics system is worth checking out.

The joy of balance training is that the process happens fast. Trainees will see results in the very first session. Depending on their age, by twelve to twenty sessions, they are at 80 percent of their potential.

It is difficult to understand this process without actually experiencing it. It is like flipping on a light switch. It is fascinating to observe people suddenly discover a capacity that they did not realize they had. Furthermore, reawakening the balance system triggers a positive feeling best described as "feeling alive." There is a sense of the whole body being activated and integrated.

Skiers know that feeling as well. If I ski all day, I know I've been depleted and worked out, but I feel more alive. I will go have dinner with my friends, and everything simply feels better. That is the sense one gets after a balance-training session. The more balance training one does, the more one's movements become increasingly fluid and athletic.

For people recovering from a concussion, the results are quite interesting. Before their first session with me, one of their symptoms is a tendency to constantly shrug their shoulders. I don't know the science behind that; it's just an observable detail. However, after balance training, the shrugging goes away.

In the next chapter, we'll look at the core principles of balance training and get a fundamental understanding of what's at work.

FALLS

I spent several weeks training with Jim and Janet in Park City over a summer but went back to New York in September with just a small foam block to practice with. One day, I foolishly climbed up on a high marble window sill in my socks to investigate a leak, and my foot slipped, sending me tumbling backward, head first toward a disastrous impact with the floor. Suddenly, I felt like I was moving in slow motion as I managed to twist myself around, break my fall by stepping on the seat of my desk chair and hitting the floor on my padded flank.

I thought it was a miracle that instead of breaking my neck, I had nothing more than a nasty black-and-blue mark on my thigh. Then, I realized it was not a miracle but the balance training that had taught me, unconsciously, how to fall without hurting myself.

— SUSAN

A heightened sense of balance can prevent falls, but I can't state unequivocally that it will prevent all falls. What it will do, however, is enable you to fall in a better, less dangerous way. When a person is in the act of falling, a good balance system kicks in to reduce the velocity of the fall so that when the body makes impact, there is less injury.

When I watch a well-balanced person fall, it is like a ballet in which the person loses balance, falls some, regains balance momentarily, falls some more, loses balance again, then regains it, over and over on the way to the ground. This cycle of losing and regaining balance slows the rate of the fall so that when the person actually does hit the ground, the speed of the fall is not so fast as to cause serious harm. The impact is lessened as a result of falling well. As counterintuitive as it sounds, better balance creates a better fall.

Part Two

===

THE BODY'S BALANCE SYSTEM

CHAPTER 5

Tools of Rebalancing

═══

CONTRALATERAL MOVEMENT

Balance, like walking and running, entails contralateral movements. When a person walks and runs, the left leg moves forward with the right hand, followed by the right leg and the left hand, and so forth. In fact, the right side of the brain controls the left side of the body and vice versa, so even the signaling from the brain is contralateral. Every athletic movement is a contralateral movement.

Some people have ipsilateral movement—the opposite of contralateral movement—in which they move with their right leg and right hand in sync. This is sometimes observable in people who are suffering from a physical illness, undergoing a great deal of stress, have a chronic disease, or are concussed.

To remedy the ipsilateral movement pattern, I will put a person through a neural reset routine, with plenty of movements crossing the body's center line. This will restore the person's natural contralateral movement.

Many weightlifting movements operate on a bilateral neural movement pattern, meaning that both sides of the body are moving simultaneously. For example, a bench press or military press requires both arms to move up and down in unison.

Athletes who have been lifting weights immediately prior to balance training see a noticeable deterioration in balance skill from previous sessions. The bilateral movements involved in weightlifting appear to reconfigure the body into the unnatural ipsilateral movement pattern and therefore, make their balance worse. I believe much of bilateral standard weightlifting like that done in deadlifts, overhead presses, Olympic lifts, and so on, may be detrimental to athletic ability if not practiced along with a strong balance-training program.

ONE LEG

Every move in any sport is performed on a single leg. Running is achieved with one foot on the ground and then the other but not both simultaneously. The act of kicking a ball involves the transference of weight from one leg to the other, with one leg firmly planting and the other swinging into a kick. Here's where things get interesting: even the act of standing is done by balancing one leg or shifting over to the other leg.

An experiment with a Ken doll or a G.I. Joe doll will demonstrate the feat that is balancing on one leg. Ken, being anatomically correct (for the purposes of the experiment anyway), is built to scale with the same proportions of a typical human body. Stand him on two feet. Sure enough, he balances and is able to stand erect.

Now bend one of those legs and have Ken balance on a single leg. Whoops, he tipped over. Maybe the other leg? Nope. It's impossible. And it's not just a problem for Ken and Joe. The entire mammalian kingdom with the exception of our species lacks this ability. In fact, everything we do is predominantly on one foot. There is no real-world scenario for two-foot balance. Every move we make involves one foot or the other bearing the brunt of the load.

With that in mind, it seems counterintuitive that we spend so much time and effort attempting to build strength in completely unnatural positions and motions, such as those used in weightlifting, which demand equal weight being borne on each foot at the same time, or arms working bilaterally rather than contralaterally.

PERIPHERAL VISION

There is a school of thought that proposes that balance training should be performed with the eyes closed, the rationale being that without the aid of sight, the subject will rely instead on only the vestibular or "pure balance" system. And this is a good idea if, and only if, one is training to be a well-balanced blind person.

This notion is constructed around a misunderstanding of the multimodalism of the balance system. The vestibular system is a singular part of a synergistic network that includes the soles of the feet, the proprioceptive sensors, the mind map, maybe the tongue, maybe the palms of the hands, and maybe some other yet-to-be-discovered part of the system. The flawed idea of a "pure" sense of balance derived from a single source disregards the multiple components operating conjunctively; therefore, shutting off an integral part in an attempt to isolate the system does not make sense.

Central vision can be over-relied upon for visual cues of alignment from the modern spaces, using the perfectly vertical and horizontal sight lines as a de facto leveling system. So in that sense, the eyes will work against better balance. Even the yoga method of focusing on a spot to help with balance is a failed precept. What I have discovered is the peripheral vision has a crucial role in the balance system and needs extensive training to engage it properly for better athletic balance. Our "river rocks" protocol offers a good example of peripheral vision's aid in balancing. When a trainee first sets foot on this re-creation of a river crossing, it is with a degree of timidity, as the eyes are focused downward. After a few attempts, however, the person is instructed to keep the head up and trust the peripheral vision. As a result, that person will handle the obstacles faster and more smoothly.

The same no-look technique applies for landing a jump or catching an object while balancing. The reality is that the eyes do see the approaching ground and do see the incoming object but just not directly. The reaction to being able to balance and catch a football without looking at it is utter surprise at first. What is happening in this act is simply the peripheral vision communicating information that a ball is coming in at such-and-such speed, trajectory, and so on, and the body naturally—autonomically—reacts to account for it.

One recent experiment involved a subject being shown a frightening image just outside the peripheral vision of which she was consciously aware. She was asked if she could see it, and of course, she couldn't. However, during the experiment her brainwaves were being measured to see if the brain was responding in any way to the fright. And sure enough, that part of her brain that would be expected to light up when seeing the image, did so despite the fact that she had no conscious awareness of having seen anything unusual. The takeaway for athletes and my observations are that there are data, as defined by Dr. Paul Bach-y-Rita, that are totally bypassing the conscious mind to the subconscious mind—the part of consciousness where you find the zone of high performance.

How is this possible? For starters, there are seven million cones in the retina. Those are the photoreceptors in the center part of the vision, detecting color and shape. Additionally, the retina contains some 120 million rods—that's roughly seventeen times more rods than cones. These rods exist in the outer rim of the retina and are so sensitive that under the right conditions, they can detect a single photon, making it about a thousand times more light-sensitive than a cone. In effect, the rods could be accessing seventeen thousand more data than the cones.

It has been argued that the purpose for these highly sensitive detectors is night vision. That might make perfect sense if humans were a nocturnal species, but we are not. So why are the rods gathering such a massive amount of information? The answer to that question appears to have some relationship to balance and our movement through the playing field and life. It also serves to demystify what is meant by expressions such as "great field vision" or "eyes in the back of his head."

Consider the elite players in basketball, baseball, football, and tennis, and how vital vision is in terms of their skill. Yes, they move with fluidity, strength, and agility, but greatness in these sports also requires incredible vision: sinking a fadeaway three-point jump shot at the buzzer; hitting a 100 mph fastball; returning a kickoff through eleven oncoming defenders for a touchdown; returning a Roger Federer serve. There is no doubt that great balance, great athletic ability, and great field awareness are inexorably linked.

Notice, by the way, that big muscles are not necessary for any of these athletic achievements. These are not mere feats of brute strength but highly developed skills. Even sports that might seem to favor big muscles may not in actuality. Many of the best fighters in the Ultimate Fighting Championship (UFC) are thin and wiry of frame. They fight differently as well, relying not on classic put-up-your-dukes tactics, but rather, on stealthy flank attacks from all angles. Defending such an attack demands sharp peripheral vision.

An example of this style of fighter is UFC champion T. J. Dillashaw, whose unconventional training methods are indicative of a new type of athlete. Among his daily activities is wakeboarding, which requires precision balance. Russell Wilson, the winning quarterback of Super Bowl XLVIII, trains on a stand-up paddleboard, which is also a challenging act of balance.

FEET

Feet are sensory devices that operate like pressure plates that collect information nanosecond by nanosecond in order to be given directions regarding placement. They go about their business rather quietly and efficiently, usually unnoticed. Still, feet are vital instruments, containing a quarter of the body's entire bones, muscles, and tendons.

Hands contain another quarter, but they are allowed to operate without the confinement that shoes necessitate. Therefore, they do not suffer the atrophying effects that feet do. Consequently, when people learn to better utilize their feet, they establish a better sense of balance.

Often, new clients will want to keep their shoes on, which makes for good contrast later on, after they realize the benefits of taking them off. But starting out, they will inevitably complain that their feet, in their overbuilt shoes begin to hurt. The reason is because they are experiencing a balance challenge, and their feet need to be involved in the process and those delicate instruments are flexing, gripping, and just working too hard to help with the balance challenge. Because they have no effect on the process through the thick soles of athletic shoes, they are overworking them, so they get tired and sore very quickly.

Eventually, the shoes come off, and *voilà!* The feet stop hurting, and balance improves for a couple of reasons. Most of the active muscles and moving parts of the foot are in the forefoot and the toes; now that they are free from the turned-up forefoot of the shoe, they can help with the balance challenge. And just as important, the hundred thousand-plus nerve sensors in foot are no longer blocked by the dulling impact of the thick soles; they can now send much better data to the balance system.

Feet are critical in the ability to balance. Research has shown that balance can be improved simply by walking on cobblestones. The first time one sets foot on cobblestones, however, it is uncomfortable, as the foot needs to adjust to the unevenness of the surface. Within moments, however, the foot morphs its musculature to adapt to the terrain it senses beneath.

STABILIZERS

Balance training also strengthens weak ankles. I can spot weak ankles during a client's first balance challenge. Some people have a history of rolling, spraining, or straining ankles. Balance training trains and builds the stabilizers throughout the total system including the lower-leg complex. After several sessions, the ankle weakness most times disappears.

Muscles function as both mobilizer and stabilizer. Mobilizer muscles are the large muscles at work in weightlifting, locomotion, and appendage movement. Stabilizer muscles, by comparison, provide precision and control. If mobilizers are the car's engine, stabilizers are the steering and suspension.

If I lift a ten-pound weight over my head with one hand, there is not much required in terms of stability. It's not terribly heavy. However, if I perform the same action with a hundred-pound weight, there's going to be some shaking as I attempt to keep my balance. The stabilizer muscles are now busy at work, controlling micromovements with rapid-fire adjustments keeping the large mobilizer muscles in place to do their job.

Balance training builds these stabilizing muscles all at once. And unlike the large muscles, which are often worked individually in isolation, the stabilizing muscles are strengthened simultaneously as a unit. Because of the nature of this training, involving so many muscles at once, even the fittest of athletes begin sweating within the first minute, often to their own surprise. They are confused because they know they are doing very little in terms of the athletic training they are used to, yet they can feel that they are getting a massive workout. Great athletes who have superior body awareness—what is called kinesthetic intelligence—know right away that what they are doing is activating muscles that are important to their success.

FALLING: A KEY TO BALANCE TRAINING?

Ironically, to improve balance, the body must approach the edge of its balance ability, a point at which anything beyond would result in a fall. This method is similar to lifting weights close to a point of failure. If all an athlete did was to challenge his or her balance by standing, then he or she would not improve his or her balance. A balance limit has to be reached to improve balance. Much of the research on improved balance and athletic ability are inconclusive because the studies require only very low-level balance challenges. Higher levels of challenges necessary for improvement could not be used because of safety concerns for the subjects and maintaining lowest common-denominator protocol across the varying levels of the subjects' balance skills. Because the subjects never had their balance seriously challenged, their balance did not get much better.

Watch young children learn how to walk. They stand up and they fall, take a few steps and they fall. They are learning how to balance by pushing their skills to the limit. This is how we train, but our methods bring the client to a point just short of a fall. We wouldn't be in business long if all of our clients fell all the time.

———

Part Three

BALANCE TO IMPROVE SPORTS PERFORMANCE

CHAPTER 6

Athletes and Bad Balance

Shannon Turley, strength and conditioning coach for Stanford's football team, reduced his team's injury rate by 87 percent between 2006 and 2012 by focusing less on raw strength and more on mobility and balance. He banned freshmen from weightlifting until they had been adequately trained in the program, and he incorporated yoga and Pilates into his regimen.

Those injury rates remain low because Turley does not have his players build strength simply for strength's sake. The body has certain power muscles, which I call mobilizer muscles. These are muscles that move body parts. When a weight is lifted, these are the muscles that are used. When an object has to be moved with greater accuracy, requiring speed and direction to be accounted for, a different type of muscle is required: the stabilizer muscles, explained in the previous chapter.

To haul my equipment, I drive a large seven thousand-pound, four hundred-horsepower diesel truck. It does not corner well, requires a long distance to stop, and although powerful, does not accelerate very well. I would love to drive a four hundred-horsepower Corvette, which can change direction like a chased jackrabbit, accelerate like a hungry cheetah, and stop on a dime. My truck has the ability to haul stuff; the Corvette has similar power but with the added dimension of control. That is what stabilizer muscles do: they provide control. They determine coordination and agility.

The danger of building only mobilizer muscles is that actions requiring strength could possibly result in injury if that strength is not properly controlled. Building large muscles without also developing the controlling stabilizing muscles has the potential for injury. What distinguishes balance training from other forms of exercise is that the former works solely on the body's stabilizer muscles.

Janet has been a successful personal trainer to athletes for twenty-five years. She has about 14 percent body fat and rides a single-speed mountain bike up the tallest mountains in Park City, Utah, often blowing by experienced riders on geared bikes.

I tell you this so you know she is clearly fit and strong. However, when she arrived to learn my balance-training system, her weak ankles were evident. She explained that she rolled her ankles frequently. They were so weak, in fact, that she could be walking down the street and her ankle would roll for no apparent reason. After fifteen sessions of balance training, Janet's ankles are now so stabilized that she has not rolled an ankle in the three-plus years since then.

Several studies report that balance training does, indeed, reduce not only ankle injuries but also hamstring and anterior cruciate ligament (ACL) injuries, among other varieties. Improving balance develops the coordination necessary to keep the body in the correct position and alignment when performing an athletic action.

Year-round weight training in sports is still a relatively new concept, and much of that weight training has not changed in decades. Sports-related injuries that are simply considered par for the course are, in my opinion, often unnecessarily suffered as a result of out-of-date training methods focusing on large, mobilizer muscles while neglecting the stabilizer muscles designed to aid in their use. In that respect, Coach Turley is on the forefront of modern conditioning, teaching his players to build *better* muscles, not *bigger* muscles.

The balance-training method I developed was originally designed to create more agile, successful athletes. However, through a series of unplanned events, I discovered that these same methods help people quickly recover from post-concussion syndrome in which the symptoms of the concussion fail to sufficiently dissipate over time. This is often a result of repeated concussions, the most dangerous forms of which are conditions called repetitive head injury syndrome and second impact syndrome (SIS). These are follow-up concussions that occur before the first concussion has had time to heal.

These follow-up concussions are often far more injurious than the initial one and can occur within hours or even a few weeks later. The repeat-concussion clients I treat, however, deal with repetitive concussions over longer periods of time. Two clients, for example, have each suffered nine concussions in a ten-year span. My conclusion is that they sustained the further injuries as a result of a lack of balance. That is to say, they believed themselves capable of athletic actions that they were, in fact, no longer able to perform as a result of having impaired their balance skills.

One of the critical tests involved in concussion protocol is designed to establish whether there has been a diminishment of balance skills. It is my contention that if the balance system is not fully reestablished, the concussion is not fully repaired. And if the balance system is out of whack, the athlete is vulnerable to yet another concussion.

There are two reasons for this assertion. First, the brain has not fully repaired itself, thus, it is more susceptible to a follow-up concussion. Second, and germane to the subject of balance, the body may not be able to adequately react in time to protect the skull.

A primary objective of the balance system is to ensure that when we fall, the autonomic body response makes every effort to protect the head first and foremost. Therefore, there is no better way to prevent the long-term repeating concussion cycle than to restore the balance system, ideally, to the highest possible level.

Humans evolved the sense of fear for a very good reason. It is one of the keys to survival, which prevented our distant ancestors from being eaten by saber-toothed tigers and other nasty predators. Fear from getting hurt was an admirable trait to possess in order to live a long life in these ancient nomadic tribes. If a reckless youth disregarded the cues from his balance system and fell, injuring his ankle to the point where he could not walk, he probably was abandoned by his nomadic tribe to die alone.

There are safer methods to improving balance than skateboarding on a half-pipe, and that is what I do with my balance-training techniques. It is possible to improve balance while honoring the fear response, and doing so will result in fewer concussions, fewer injuries—career-ending or otherwise—and will ultimately create better athletes.

My method of training respects that when it comes to improving balance, the human body performs best at its own individual pace. We don't post motivational posters on the walls that speak of ignoring pain or disregarding fear, nor do we yell and exhort our clients to push past their limits.

The CDC estimates that 1.6 to 3.8 million concussions occur annually in sports and recreational activities. Other reporting puts the number of hospital visits at 275,000 at a cost of $60 billion. Head protection can, to some extent, help reduce this problem, but better balance restoration and improved post-concussion health also factor in significantly.

Whether jogging or skateboarding, dedicated balance training will aid in injury prevention—not necessarily by preventing all falls, but by improving the ability to reduce the impact of a fall. Every nanosecond counts in the act of falling, as the body is repositioned on its way to the ground. Watching how a person falls reveals volumes about that person's balance ability.

The best balanced athletes are the most coordinated and agile athletes in their sport. These athletes have some of the very best situational awareness and are in the perfect state of flow. They also are able to use their strength to its fullest capability and have fewer injuries. In the following chapters I will review how each of these happens by virtue of simply improving your balance.

CHAPTER 7

Agility

===

Dictionaries define *agility* as the ability to move quickly and easily. For my purposes, a deeper understanding is required. Agility is the ability to control and operate one's body at high speed, under stress, and in space.

Coordination is a component of agility. Coordination zeroes in on body control. A golfer, who doesn't have to defend Kobe Bryant on a basketball court, does not need great agility to win the Masters. However, he does require coordination.

To return to the idea of defending a great basketball player like Kobe Bryant, the task demands great agility, which is necessitated by great coordination. Thus, when we speak of an athlete as being agile, it goes without saying that he is also very coordinated.

There is at least a sense that the most agile and well-coordinated athlete is generally the best athlete on the field. I would predict that in pro soccer or any sport, the most coordinated and agile athletes are also the most successful players. They can maintain control of their body and movements at high speed while confronting various challenges in the course of play: dribbling at full speed, stopping abruptly, quick changes of direction, opposing players getting in their way, and so on. The most agile player can obviously respond better than a less agile athlete.

So where does balance come in? When you listen to sportscasters describe a professional athlete as having "great balance," it remains an ethereal and somewhat fuzzy word. As agility relates to balance, consider the following equation:

$$COORDINATION + AGILITY = BALANCE$$

What do I mean by "equal" in the above equation? If you add 1 point to each side of an equation, the equation remains equal. This means that if I raise balance 1 point, I've raised agility and coordination 1 point. You can flip the equation around, of course:

$$BALANCE = COORDINATION + AGILITY$$

So, when an athlete improves balance, his or her balance ability, coordination, and agility are resultantly improved to the same extent. Because these skills encompass a wide variety of athletic activities, they are not easily turned into quantifiable metrics. A more commonly understood athletic value, on the other hand, is strength.

It is easy enough for most people to lift a five-pound weight a dozen times without any real effort. So, if that person spent three days a week for eight weeks lifting that five-pound weight a dozen times, no strength will be gained. The only way to progress is to infuse classic principles of training progression: either by increasing the number of reps or sets, increasing the amount of weight, or decreasing the amount of rest between sets. These variables help increase the stress through which the body responds by becoming stronger.

Apply that line of thought into the balance equation. Recall that the limit of one's balance ability is defined by the working limit of the subconscious ANS system, that is, one can only move as quick and as fast as his or her body will allow. Thus, if a lack of balance is preventing a reserve of muscle and strength from being accessed, then that potential will not be realized. On the other hand, improving that balance ability will unlock those reserves, in turn, creating better athleticism.

Improving balance, therefore, acts as a key in unlocking stored potential. Additionally, improving balance improves the kinetic chain, allowing the body to become more graceful and athletic. This is demonstrable in the improvements to vertical leap. Better balance activates an entire system, putting it suddenly online. The body is now able to tap into previously dormant potential, wasted strength in this case, and draw upon it to achieve a higher upward jump.

The same thing is true with hitting a ball, whether it be in tennis, golf, baseball, or any other similar sport. Rigidity of movement results in less power, which translates in tennis as, among other weaknesses, a slower serve, in golf as a shorter drive, and in baseball as a routine grounder or pop fly. However, that tightness can be eliminated through balance training, with the result that the kinetic chain can be lit up, igniting greater access to power.

The NFL Combine (an annual scouting event showcasing the athletic skills of an incoming class of potential recruits) is a case study in balance evaluation. Scouts measure agility and coordination through a shuttle-run drill known as the cone drill or the 5-10-5, which measures lateral quickness. Beginning in a three-point stance, the athlete explodes five yards to the right, taps a line, then hustles back ten yards to his left, touches another line, then pivots and runs five more yards to the finish, ideally, in under seven seconds.

During a year in which I studied the combine, I looked at what this test meant in a real sense for the highly skilled position of wide receiver. The highest-paid receiver garnered a contract of $5 million a year. The next tier of receivers earned $1 million annually. After that, the money dropped off significantly. A look at their cone drill performances reveals that tenths-of-a-second equated to millions of dollars.

When one considers the wider world of sports, it becomes apparent just how valuable—in a literal sense—balance improvement can be. Improved balance improves both agility and coordination, and furthermore, it unlocks unused power, speed, strength, endurance, stamina, flexibility, accuracy, and more.

COORDINATION + AGILITY = BALANCE

To get a better handle on how this works, the next chapter is devoted to coordination.

CHAPTER 8

Coordination: The Fluidity in Great Balance

A discussion about coordination needs to begin with what it is that we need to coordinate, namely, the kinetic chain of the movement we want to improve. Coordination is especially crucial to highly prized skills, such as throwing, striking, or shooting.

There's currently a very popular term in use, particularly among personal trainers and at gyms: *kinetic chain*. Ask around the training world, and you'll likely get a variety of definitions about what it is. The reason for that probably has a lot to do with the definition of word *kinetic* itself: it means "of, or relating to motion, or the result of motion." So, roughly speaking, *kinetic theory* is essentially the collective knowledge about how components of matter operate when the body is in motion.

Another term arises in discussions about kinetic chain and that is *biomechanics*. If you're moving well throughout the kinetic chain, it's likely you're going to be described as having good biomechanics.

There's going to be plenty of nuance involved in defining the kinetic chain and a lot of debate as a result. The same is true of biomechanics, but for our purposes, let's keep things simple. The human body is a super complex system of systems, from nerves to muscles to senses to fascia to joints to metabolism, and so on and so forth, and the more efficiently all of those systems work with one another to achieve an athletic objective, the better the athlete.

OK, so for every movement (athletic or otherwise), there has to be a series of coordinated muscle-firing patterns happening in an organized way. If I'm a golfer, I'm going to draw my club back and get this whole system coiled up with potential energy. Then I have to uncoil the hip, then the shoulder, then the arms, then the club, and the club face comes through. What if I get that club up, uncoil the shoulder first, and I come through with the hip later than I ideally should? Of course, that's going to be a bad golf shot.

For an optimal athletic movement, everything has to fire in an organized, controlled way. A great golf swing is often described as being "fluid," and that's a good way to describe a well-oiled system of motor patterns, with muscles firing in the proper order. Another good word to use here is "coordination," which, of course, is what we're trying to dig into with this chapter.

Tension is a killer when it comes to the coordinated sequence of a good athletic movement. Tension inhibits the kinetic chain, but that tension can be reduced by strengthening the stabilizer muscles.

Imbalances within the muscle-firing patterns often lead to poor coordination of the kinetic chain of a movement. If I have an overdeveloped set of quadriceps and I have underdeveloped hamstrings, it's going to affect my performance. I'm not able to utilize all of the strength buried in those fibers because of the conflict and overdevelopment. The hamstrings, for example, are not being used to their fullest potential because of the overly powered quadriceps; they have to work harder to do their job.

This results in a misfire of the kinetic chain. Power is lost or gets choked up in the process, and in the end, you have a retarded movement. Athletic potential is not being fully deployed.

When we do balance training, we want to activate all parts of the body. The essence of balance training is that you have to learn how to use all the muscles with good coordination—coordinated through the ideal kinetic chain of the movement.

When we train balance at our facility in Park City, we find people who will have different comments about which part of the body they feel is being affected in the session. "I feel that in my hips," "I feel that in my calf muscle," or "I feel it in my back." What these identifications usually mean is that we've discovered a weakness or misalignment in that location of the kinetic chain.

Dana Santas, the developer of the athletic performance yoga method, Radius Yoga, had a party and put ten of her MLB trainers clients and friends on her SlackBow. My balance training invention. They didn't seem particularly interested in the big-picture approach to balance but instead focused on how the SlackBow exposed the weak links in their kinetic chain. I think that is because they intuitively know that if they fix that hot spot, the flow of power—through the kinetic chain—is going to improve their players' performance. Go to slackbow.com/science to read Dana's brilliant and scientific take on why this happens on a SlackBow.

The coordination of the kinetic chain is the key to success in every sport you can think of. Strength alone is not enough; the muscles firing in a perfectly organized way makes the difference.

Balance training seeks to train all the super subtle wirings and firings of your physical and mental systems, with the coordination of the kinetic chain being a primary beneficiary of the work.

CHAPTER 9

Hitting and Striking With Accuracy and Strength

Striking with accuracy and power—coordination and control of movement—is critical. How can balance training help us master this?

Every golfer who has been trained using my methods, quickly, within a few sessions, is hitting the ball farther and with more accuracy. When a golfer swings his club, he has to coordinate and control many different forces to bring the clubface back to the ball with power and the perfect angle to make a good shot. If he swings harder than what he can control, he will lose his balance ever so slightly and mishit the ball.

To keep this from happening, he must slow down his swing to control the clubhead better. Try it yourself; go swing a club as hard as you can, and you will clearly throw your body off-balance. The formula is so simple: improve balance and one can swing the club with more speed and create longer shots.

There is pretty good research that PGA golfers have considerably better balance than high-ranking amateurs. When you see how fast a PGA player swings his club, you also sense that he has incredible balance to be able to handle those forces. Among athletes I train, pro golfers have some of the best balance.

All the positions one needs to be in during the swing can be held with better balance. This is a recurring theme through this and the next two chapters. Anytime a force is being created by the body to swing, hit, or throw, the body must be able to control those forces, otherwise accuracy is lost. Everyone knows that in general, to be more accurate, you swing easier. Why? To keep those forces under control.

Think of the tennis player. There is a huge amount of force coming through when she swings the racquet—just a storm of force. So she needs to be able to control her body or she is going to hit the ball wrong by a fraction of a fraction of what is needed to deliver the ball to a targeted location on the other side of the court.

A revealing aspect about sports in which striking with power and accuracy is involved is apparent in the way that performance can differ from one day to the next. Think about the batter in baseball who is on fire one day but can't seem to catch a break the next. A lot of variables are in play, for certain, one of which can be the state of balance. If balance is a bit off, and the coordination of the kinetic chain is off along with it, the fluid stream of power is disrupted. Things don't connect, including the ability to put a bat on a ninety-five-mile-per-hour fastball.

Perhaps this idea is best illustrated in golf. Whereas with a batter, a different pitcher might make a huge difference in his effectiveness, in golf, it's just the player, the ball, the clubs, the course, and the weather. One day, he blasts each drive three hundred yards down the middle of every fairway. The next day, he may not have the same distance or accuracy.

The reason for the difference might be that he is neurologically organized a little differently today than yesterday. I've got everything lined up for a shot, perfectly aligned over the ball. Somewhere in the swing, the body changes by thousandths of an inch, resulting in a change in the clubhead path, generating a ten-meter change in the direction the ball flies off the face of the club.

Another problem is over-swinging to today's balance level. Let's go back to the batter in the box, wanting to swing hard at a pitch. An over-swing will cause him to lose balance—same thing with golf. What I want to do is to stay within the neurological limit of that control and coordination—balance. Increase your balance, and your power can be opened up. But it won't look hard: a well-oiled kinetic chain in which all the systems are in sync and moving together fluidly and in proper sequence makes it look easy.

CHAPTER 10

Throwing With Accuracy and Strength

If you're striking, you are using rotational force: you come through with the punch, and you've got to hold that force as it comes through. Throwing is similar. I think of throwing and striking as being very similar in terms of balance and coordination.

With throwing, every type of throw that I make requires that I rotate. Consider a pitcher. He stands on his back leg, turns his body sideways to home plate, rotates even further with his back almost to the pitcher, then with controlled violent coordination, he unfurls this kinetic chain with a massive rotational move toward the plate so that all the force he can muster is imparted into the ball. For a fraction of a second, his left leg must hold all of these forces in place just as he releases the ball. If the left leg loses its position for just a second, then the pitch will not go where he wants. Our pitching clients are always amazed that they have better balance on their left leg. About 98 percent of all our new clients come in with better balance on their left leg. For right-handed people, it is the landing leg for all rotational moves: hitting, swinging, throwing, and kicking.

Whether throwing a discuss 240 feet or sailing a football 40 yards down the field into the clutches of a speeding receiver, everything has to be on a point of balance for the sake of that rotation and control of the force within that rotation. If the athlete throws harder than his balance has the capacity to maintain, the throw will be off, fall short, and he may even fall over.

Balance, coordination, and the resulting control of movement allow an athlete to throw with power and hit the target.

CHAPTER 11

Aiming and Targeting

———

Balance training can also improve aiming skills.

A forty-five-year-old professional golfer stands over his ball getting ready to make a putt eight feet from the hole. He has made this same putt hundreds of times before. He sees the break and his line perfectly. Confidently, he stands over the ball, draws back his putter, strikes the ball perfectly only to see it slide just past the hole.

"How could this be?" he thinks to himself. "I hit it perfectly. I know I had the line just right." Then he thinks, "I never missed these when I was younger."

For a minute, let's analyze the golfer. Putting does not

take strength, so age-related strength loss it not a factor. He recently had Lasik surgery, so vision loss is not a factor. He has practiced putting five days a week for the last twenty-five years, so theoretically, the more someone does something, the better he or she should get. What could have gone wrong?

Here is what happened. He stands over the ball and everything is perfectly aligned, including his mind and confidence. As he pulls his club back, his body position changes by just a minuscule imperceptible amount which will take the putter off his intended line by a fraction of a millimeter. That small change is just enough to change the direction of the ball so that it misses the cup. As we age, without balance training, our balance ability will decline, and therefore, we then lose the ability to hold perfectly still.

The term for it is *postural sway*. To stand perfectly still, the balance system has to be highly tuned. Hundreds of muscles work together to keep us standing still. The balance system coordinates this massive symphony of control. This is why young golfers stand over a putt and without much thought, jam the ball in the hole. Because of the weaker balance system in the older golfer, he may be more balanced one day than the next. His ball striking will be inconsistent, causing him to wonder why he hit it so well yesterday but not today.

One of the problems is postural sway, which is difficult to recognize because the decline is so small. However, a putt does not need any more than a small fraction of a millimeter in the clubface alignment to make a difference.

The same is true for shooters, archers, pool players, and darts players. We have a client who is an Olympic-style shooter. A perfect score in this style of shooting is 200. When he first came in, his personal best was 165. After two sessions, his personal best jumped to 172. Four more sessions after that, he jumped to 181. I don't know anything about Olympic-style shooting, but I was told that the typical improvement rate is a point here and there and that at his level, large jumps in personal best are unheard of.

When lining up a shot to pull the trigger, any postural sway will cause the bullet or pellet to miss its mark by quite a bit.

To hold one's position perfectly still to shoot a rifle or a bow takes a well-balanced system. To hold one's position through a golf swing, throwing a dart, or even a free throw is also an act of balance. Or at least being able to do it constantly well is a balance skill. I believe that putting well one day but not the next is mostly caused by poor balance. Those who are consistently good have better balance.

CHAPTER 12

Running

KINETIC CHAIN-OF-BALANCE RUNNING

When we talk about running—about enjoying running, about good mechanics, about reducing injuries, and about running well (be that longer, faster, or both)—a sincere discussion has to drill down into the topic of the kinetic chain. A highly functioning kinetic chain in running means that all of the muscles are firing in the proper order. It means the arms and legs are working harmoniously so that a dynamic state of balance is achieved and maintained as the body hurtles through space in a perpetual state of falling forward but without falling over.

As natural as running is to us as bipedal humans, it's a complicated affair. Engineers can build a ship and guide it to Pluto, but when it comes to building a robot that can run, the balance problem makes for a billion-dollar headache. It took a lot of scientific innovation to build the Boston Dynamics robot that is close but still far away from how a human runs. The engineering problems involved in keeping a robot in balance one foot at a time (which is the same for us) are enormous. Now think about what's involved in running on a flat road. Then think about what's involved in running on a rocky trail with streams and roots to navigate.

In working on the running performance of a human being, an improved sense of balance will improve that kinetic chain. At its most basic level, running is a sequence of balance shifts—from being balanced on one foot to being balanced on the other, over and over. With that image in mind, think about how much energy goes into maintaining balance while simply standing on one foot—standing and balancing on one foot, not going anywhere, requires that I engage the complete balance system. If I don't have good balance, then just standing on one foot is difficult, and I'm limited in what I can do. Improve balance, and those limits dissolve.

The same is true with running. If I improve my sense of balance, the kinetic chain efficiency improves. When that happens, less energy and muscular activity are required throughout the run. I become more efficient. This applies whether I'm sprinting one hundred meters or tramping one hundred miles through the mountains.

There is even a bigger value for balance in running: energy conservation and fewer injuries. If I stand on one foot, I have to engage the balance system to keep from falling over. The worse your balance, the more energy you will have to spend to keep steady. If I have good balance, I will be able to stand on one foot without swaying left and right, forward and back. Running is similar to standing on one foot in that it is an activity performed on a single foot at a time.

If I'm running and just for a split second I begin to lose balance, think about the loss. I have to use an energy component to regain balance for that split second. Multiply that by the 1,064 steps it takes to complete a mile at six-minute pace. That is a significant use of energy that might be better applied toward other things. In a long run or race, it is a gaping hole in efficiency. In a short race, it can be the difference between first and last.

Researchers have found that those runners who run in a wider foot-stride pattern are not as efficient. It is my contention that they run in a wider foot-stride pattern because it is the more balanced position for them. More-efficient runners tend to run on a more narrow strike pattern. It makes sense, of course: a wider stance leads to more balance, whereas a narrow stance has less inherent stability to it.

The narrow stride is more fruitful in terms of covering ground quickly because with the wider stance, a person is having to spend energy to go directions that aren't perfectly straight forward. Energy is wasted as the body moves in a side-to-side motion and not a 100-percent-forward motion. The result is that you're spending extra energy to go side to side.

ATHLETE ALL DAY LONG—EVEN AT WORK

One piece of advice I have for runners and all athletes for that matter is that they pay attention to how they move and the quality of their form—not just when they're out logging their daily run but also throughout the day.

If you have remastered your running so that you don't heel strike, and you use good posture and overall biomechanics, take and apply that awareness with you throughout the day. While walking, learn to land on your forefoot rather than lazily landing on your heels. Rather than walking stiff legged, emulate the relaxed, agile athlete with the head up, the knees bent, and a springy gait. Even while standing, see if you can get out of the locked-knee, weight-on-our-heels stance. Put your weight on the forefoot, scrunch your big toe to activate it, wake it up so to speak, and slightly bend your knees.

The Tarahumara are a Native American people of northwestern Mexico, renowned for their long-distance running ability. They teach their young children how to develop a feel for running on a trail by having the kids run and kick a rock down a trail without looking at the rock directly. It's a technique to tune the peripheral vision and the overall balance system into autonomously doing the navigation work for you.

Trail runners can easily apply this technique. Keep the head and eyes up while running, and let the autonomic nervous system (ANS) light up your balance system. This is how I teach people to walk and run on trails. Keep your head up. That said, I want you to look down when your instinct says to look down, because that's your peripheral vision doing a check. You check, and you look back up again. If you run with your head constantly down, you'll never succeed.

I'm a big fan of trail running, by the way. Walking and running on trails and being outdoors is emotionally beneficial, clears the brain, and gives the mood a burst of positive energy. The world of uneven surfaces triggers a defocusing reaction. It also makes for better runners because there is no way to heel strike while running up and down uneven trails. The only form you can execute on a hilly uneven trail is the correct form.

BAREFOOT RUNNING

Near where I live in Park City, we have a restaurant operated by a woman from Mexico's Copper Canyon, a place made famous in the book *Born to Run*. She used to have a pair of the authentic running sandals that were described in the book—the footwear of choice of the Tarahumara, the inexhaustible ultrarunning tribe featured in the book. The shoes are no longer there, but I saw them. Made from tires, they just hang on your feet with a couple of leather strings.

I bring this up because one thing that becomes clear about the Tarahumara is this: they weren't all actually running barefoot. They had protection underneath their feet. Even the character Barefoot Ted was running with a minimalist shoe, the Vibram.

My point about barefoot running is that we live in a world of concrete and various hard and unnatural surfaces. We also have weather to contend with. The Native Americans wore shoes at certain times of the year. Granted, they were just skins on the bottom of the feet, but that allows for another valuable insight: I think the thing that can make shoes destructive to your feet (and, of course, to your balance) is the construction of the shoe. Overbuilt shoes change the way you interact with the ground, atrophy the many powers of the foot, and intrude on how your foot senses the ground (a cornerstone of balance).

Therefore, the less material, the better. The ideal shoe would have enough tread for basic traction and protection, but that's it. I have no problem if you're running on a trail that you use a little heavier tread. But I think that the toes ought to be as free and open as possible. I am a fan of a wider toe box even in a ski boot. Free, active toes help with balance.

In my wide toe-box shoes, my toes move like crazy. I think wide toe-box shoes are important. Going barefoot is fine if you want to do it, but you would have to go to work barefoot to make that of any value. That is, you have to toughen your feet up through a lengthy and patient progression. It is not an overnight process.

The same is true with minimalistic shoes. You have to take time to adapt your mobility, ankle flexion, and foot strength so that you don't get hurt. Your feet can adapt to just about anything you throw at them if you give them time.

INJURY PREVENTION WITH BETTER BALANCE

Balance training is not going to erase the potential for running-related injuries. There are always going to be risks, and running injuries can be produced by a variety of different factors. First and foremost among these factors is that it involves doing one repetitive cycle of one cyclical motion in one direction and one plane of movement. It's a recipe for wearing things out. That said, an improvement in balance, which is expressed through better agility, coordination, and awareness, can help a runner prevent injuries.

I stated above that better runners have a narrower stride and that this is more efficient. I believe the wider more-inefficient stride is also cause for injury. The wider stride will cause unnatural lateral forces on the ankles, knees, and hips. These joints are not made for constant repetitive lateral forces. This constant pounding of lateral forces can't be good for these joints.

There has been some research suggesting that balance training will reduce injuries in sports. What's the difference being made? It comes down to the mobilizer muscles to move me forward in space. If my balance is out of tune, every time that I am foot striking, my stabilizer muscles are not fully engaged, not being used properly. It could be just a fraction of additional stress on a tendon or a knee cap, or there might be a misalignment, resulting in cartilage wear on the knee or the ankle.

FALLING TO RUN BETTER

Also, learning how to use your feet and having a sense of what your feet are doing improve the foot strike by encouraging a better landing position.

Running-form expert Dr. Nicholas Romanov is a physicist and understands the nature of balance in regard to running. He starts his lectures reminding people that gravity has everything to do with how we run. Gravity is the force that draws us into falling forward. Romanov's running technique is basically a series of controlled falls, foot to foot to foot to foot.

You are landing on a pod of sensors that are telling you where you are in space. Romanov is an advocate for minimalistic shoes and strong, mobile feet. By allowing a foot to be a foot, and for the sensory mechanisms to communicate fully and freely, you can get a lot out of your sense of balance.

The more attuned the sensors of the foot are, the more well balanced the landing position, and the less likely the possibility of injuries.

CHAPTER 13

Field Awareness

Great athletes have great field awareness. They make no-look passes, they "sense" when a defender is approaching, and they see a play or move occurring seconds before it actually happens.

Watch a great NBA point guard dribble down the court on a fast break, make a crazy move, pump fake in one direction, and throw a no-look pass the opposite direction. How did he do all that? The player who has the best court awareness is generally the best athlete on the court, and that tends to hold true sport by sport.

Russell Wilson, the Super Bowl-winning quarterback, has great field awareness. A great quarterback can look down the field and see how all the defenders and receivers are going through their moves to either defend or catch a ball and then at just the right time, the quarterback will throw the ball perfectly to his receiver. Wilson does that one better. He does all of the above, plus he has the peripheral vision to sense when a defender has him in his sights. Watch Wilson, he will be moving out of the pocket, and a defender will launch off his feet or make his final step to tackle Wilson. At the last second, without so much as looking or even acknowledging the tackler has launched, Wilson, almost nonchalantly, takes a small step, and the attacker flies by him giving him another split second to complete his pass.

The same could be said for an elite-level ballerina or a black belt martial artist who can see everything within sight and react to it with lightning speed. Field awareness begins by practicing non-focused vision—taking in the entire landscape with the full range of deep vision, rather than locking in on one item and acting on it in a conscious manner.

As we mentioned before with our river rocks routines, the clients want to look down throughout the exercise. That downward stare locks them into a conscious mind type of thinking which causes them to move awkwardly through our artificial river crossing. We then instruct them to do the exercise with their head and eyes up using their peripheral vision.

When they lift their head and eyes up, they begin to get the hang of it, tensions drip away, the mind goes quiet, and they start to move in an athletic fashion with an explosive motion. The client is increasing his field awareness, as a function of rebooting the autonomous sense of balance to do the hard work for him. Good field awareness like good balance means trusting one's peripheral vision.

CHAPTER 14

Gravity Sports, Your Speed Limit

I've said earlier that skiing is one of the sports in which good balance is at a premium. Skiing speed depends on balance level to a great extent, because the fear or discomfort one feels is the autonomous nervous system saying, "You don't have the tools to ski this fast on a slope this difficult and stay upright."

But as you work on your balance, both your speed and control improve almost as if it is magic. You, of course, can improve your skiing ability and balance on the slope, but because the cost of failure is so high—for example, hitting a tree or breaking a leg—only small incremental improvements will occur on the slope. One of the great things about our balance-training program, as opposed to trying to improve your balance on the ski run, is that with safe protocols and progression, the cost of failure is nearly zero.

We challenge our clients' balance with incremental increases. Once we get to that new level, we confront them with a new challenge, followed by another. The cost of failure throughout this entire process is nearly zero. In this environment, we can move clients faster through each cycle of balance improvement. Attempting to improve balance through the regular practice of most sports moves at a crawl because the cost of failure requires moving forward at a much slower pace.

Janet rides a single-speed mountain bike. So when she rides downhill, she does not have any gears to switch into in order to pedal faster. She will tell you that after several sessions of balance training, her downhill speeds increased dramatically. The only thing she added to her fitness regimen was balance training. Better balance allows Janet to enter turns and negotiate rough rocky sections at a faster speed thus improving her overall downhill speed.

For skiers, incorporating balance work helps with longevity. In fact, my original purpose in designing the SlackBow Balance Training program was so that I could ski—and ski fast—when I am ninety. I believe that many skiers, except those lucky enough to ski every day, stop skiing because their balance declines when it does not have to. I have been skiing for sixty years and know it does not take much skill or strength to ski down an intermediate run. Balance decline causes the skier to be more and more cautious until it is no longer fun so he quits skiing all together.

In the 2014 Olympics, I paid a lot of attention to the skiers, particularly their balance. A skier with good balance whom I watched was thirty-six-year-old Bode Miller, the winningest American skier ever in his final Olympics.

In the downhill competition, there are three practice runs followed by a single run that counts. In his trio of training runs, Miller placed first, sixth, and first. He killed it in the training runs, appearing loose with his upper body to make millions of microcorrections along the way.

Then came the race. Miller's arms were stiff and did not move like they did in the training runs. What that tells me is that he was not fully utilizing his balance system. One of the most important requirements of skiing fast is to keep the skis on the snow. If the skis bounce off even for a millisecond, the skier loses speed. The way to keep your skis on the snow is to absorb each and every one of the millions of balance challenges with a supple body.

The outcome was that Miller finished eighth. He blamed the weather conditions and the course for his performance. I won't doubt him, and I am sure that if he says they were factors, then they were. But I saw something else. I think what happened is that the pressure may have caused him to try too hard, to try to control the race consciously rather than allowing himself to enter a flow state to handle the complex mechanisms of balance necessary for skiing a downhill race.

Younger skiers, snowboarders, and surfers are often characterized as being fearless. I see this fearlessness as a sign of their youthful high balance skills. However, there will be a slight decay in the sense of balance for an aging athlete, a skill that an athlete from any of these sports can improve in the safety of a gym.

I think that in Bode's case, he had undergone a miniscule degradation in balance, which affects all aging athletes. At thirty-six, Miller was clearly as strong as he was when he was twenty-six. He has a phenomenal fitness program. I certainly don't think his skill level had deteriorated. If anything, given his experience and high intelligence, he was at the zenith of skiing skill level. Just a small loss of balance skills may have been the difference.

There is not yet a method of measuring the highest levels

of athletic balance. If there was a measure, then an athlete like Miller could test to see if he had a slight loss of balance skills and work to get them back. In this book, I have mentioned the Klopman Balance Index (KBI)—the 0-100 scale, ranging from no balance to the very best balance in the world. The KBI could be such a tool, but at this time, the problem is that I am currently the only one who knows how to use it. We have filed a patent and are currently working on digitizing the KBI so that maybe soon, we can have a product for the rest of the world to use.

CHAPTER 15

Balance Creates the Hard-to-Achieve Flow

When we train our clients in balance training, there is no background music on, and we don't allow them to wear headphones. Research, of course, indicates that people can lift more weight with music playing. And research might eventually prove that subjects can balance better with music playing. The problem is that music acts as an artificial way of shutting off the conscious mind and allowing the body to achieve the state of flow necessary to maintain good balance. Improving balance will improve your mind's ability to focus, so it is best to turn off the artificial means of shutting off your conscious mind.

Michael was a client who enjoyed paddleboard racing. But as good as he was, he had a problem of losing his balance during races. He came to me for help. In the gym, he had the best balance of any client I had. He was even better than I. After several sessions, I was feeling confident that he was going to do great in his next race. Nope, he did terribly! He fell off his board too many times to mention. I was confused. Then I realized he always balance trained with his headphone in his ears listening to music. I had asked him several times to not use the music but to no avail. When we got back to training after his disastrous race, I suggested he get a waterproof case for his iPod and listen to music during his next race. Easy to see where this story ends up. He did great in his next race.

When the balance system is operating at its maximum level of performance, there is almost no capacity left for conscious thought. The conscious mind has to be clear to reach that level. When a client is doing a balance challenge and he does something that requires conscious thought—evaluating his performance, for example—he will inevitably lose his balance within a few seconds. The same is true if he considers a compliment. That tiny bit of conscious thought is enough to reorient his mind out of the zone and back into the conscious area, which results in a loss of balance.

As clients improve their balance, they find this state of flow easier to achieve. The explanation for this is still not known, but looking at the best athletes in the world, there does seem to exist a connection between balance and concentration.

CHAPTER 16

Concussion Repair and Prevention

THE NEED FOR BALANCE

Several years ago, after spending a large amount of money on one of the nation's leading psychiatrists and failing to get better, I was at my wits' end. He was the last of several I had over forty years. I'd read what seems like thousands of self-help books. Needless to say, I did not feel like I was making any headway with my issues. One of the books was authored by Dr. Daniel Amen, who also had a series on public TV and a TED talk, and who has written many books about the brain. He is a one-man army in the fight for better brain health. After years of people telling me

I needed to get my head examined, I decided to do just that and have it examined by Dr. Amen.

Dr. Amen's clinic did a brain single-photon emission computed tomography (SPECT) scan on me, and they said, "You've got the brain of a professional football player." I had a lot of damage. I was shocked. I did not want to believe it. It took nine months for the information to finally sink in.

The photo below is a SPECT scan. The scan represents brain activity. It is not an image of tissue. The missing parts are nonfunctioning tissue. The image on the left is a healthy brain; the one on the right is mine. The prefrontal cortex is at the top of the image, and the cerebellum is at the bottom.

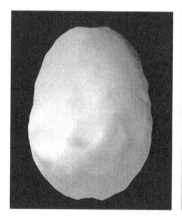 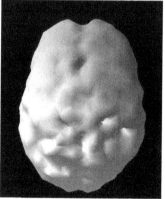

It occurred to me that I have always had a fascination with balance. For years, the only place that I ever felt comfortable and peaceful was on a ski hill, racing down at ridiculously high speeds. And that happens to be one of the greatest balance challenges of all. If it wasn't skiing, it was some other balance challenge. I have felt this way with any sport that involves speed and balance.

The brain scans revealed that I had suffered considerable damage in the cerebellum. My working theory is that that some kind of trauma occurred at a very young age. Other areas that were affected were clearly due to concussions that I had sustained through the years as a result of thrill seeking and being a little bit out of control.

Dr. Amen's team told me that my cerebellum was damaged, and one of the remedies was neuroplastic repair. While it is hard to repair the actual tissue, they explained that other parts of the brain could be trained to take over the responsibilities of the part that was damaged. And that's when they told me I needed to do balance training.

I explained that I already did balance training. They said I needed to do more. I told them they didn't understand—I balance-train people for a living. They assured me that I still needed to do more. I wasn't about to tell them that I was sure I had the best balance system of any sixty-year-old in the country.

I soon discovered that my fascination with balance work, skiing, and other balance-necessary sports had a purpose. I was actually healing my brain. Even as a teenager, I was seeking relief.

After that discussion with the doctor, I started reading all I could about concussions and traumatic brain injuries (TBIs). Balance, I learned, is one of the key tests used to assess a TBI. The best method is to get a baseline balance score prior to performing a sport and then measuring your score after sustaining a hit to the head. If the score is lower, it is a sign of a concussion.

"So if that's the case," I thought, "perhaps the reverse is also true—that improving balance will improve brain health." That was my hypothesis, which I mentioned to a client, a speech physical therapist for stroke victims. As fate seemed to have it, her son, a terrific football player, had recently suffered his third major concussion. She told me that he was done with football.

After a couple of weeks, his symptoms were still present, and he showed no signs of getting better. His mother called me and requested that I work with him. After just six sessions, his symptoms vanished. It was evident that the balance work triggered some sort of self-repair. I attribute some of that healing to simply rebooting the neurological system, but another factor is neuroplastic repair.

NEUROPLASTICITY AND NEUROREHABILITATION

Neuroplastic repair is the process where the brain reassigns functions from a damaged part of the brain to a healthy part. For example, when a stroke victim loses the function of his left arm from damage in the part of his brain that controls the left arm, his physical therapy will be to work with the left arm to function again. As his left arm function returns, his brain reassigns the left arm control to another part of the brain.

At the University of Wisconsin's Tactile Communication and Neurorehabilitation Laboratory (TCNL), they have developed the Portable Neuromodulation Stimulator (PoNS) device. The PoNS sensor is placed in the mouth to stimulate the nerves of the tongue. The idea is that lingual stimulation combined with therapeutic exercise enables the brain to form new neural pathways. This is used to recover motor functions, such as balance and movement, in not only people affected by stroke, but also in people affected by multiple sclerosis (MS), cerebral palsy, TBIs, and Parkinson's disease.

The researchers at TCNL believe that the PoNS device is effective because the tongue has a very high concentration of nerves and is connected to large, important neural pathways in the neck.

Our balance-training methods result in a massive neural stimulation of the entire body's nervous system, essentially doing the same thing as the PoNS device except that it is throughout the whole body. Our results are often similar to that of the PoNS device results. Additionally, we also see a similar pattern of positive results falloff after early sessions.

After successfully treating my high school football player client, I went a whole year without receiving any more concussion patients. Then, representatives from a local brain trauma clinic visited me. I explained my methods and theories about recovery, and they began sending me their problematic clients.

The first was a TBI patient from the University of Alaska. She had post-concussion syndrome in which the symptoms did not resolve. She could no longer ride a bike or ski, had reading problems, and experienced cognitive and anxiety issues. My observation was that she had movement patterns typical of people who have suffered brain injuries.

After her third session, she told me that she was training with a vision specialist. After her fourth session, I had to find out what the vision training involved. She produced a document that looked like a page of random letters. The exercise was to find the hidden alphabet in sequence "A, B, C," and so forth. I asked her to show me. She found the sequence and began to read it, getting to "K." She stopped, stunned, and told me that she had never gotten farther than "C" until then.

She showed me another test. This one was supposed to be completed in thirty seconds or less. Her record was beyond ninety seconds. I had her take it. She finished in under thirty seconds. Her vision therapist told her that it would take six weeks to get her time to under thirty seconds, but here she was, way ahead of schedule, having just completed her balance challenges.

I had a business associate named Bob who asked me if I worked with MS patients. I told him I had one with mild symptoms. Bob asked me if I would meet with his wife, Catie, which I did. When she walked in for her appointment, I began to second-guess myself. She came in leaning on Bob and on a cane. She felt very uncomfortable walking. I did not have the nerve to tell her that her condition was too acute that she should see a physical therapist. I adjusted the usual protocol, and we did our first session sitting down.

Catie not only had MS, but she also had nerve damage and acute pain in her pelvis from a botched surgery. She had been doing physical therapy for a long time and had really worked at getting better. After six sessions, she was amazed at her progress. I, too, am still amazed when I see how rapidly improvement happens. It feels like magic.

There is an inner drive to reboot the balance system. That has been borne out by own personal experience as well. I believe this relates to our innate human desire to have our balance challenged, as the result is euphoric, like the release of endorphins. It makes us feel good to go out in nature, see fractal surfaces, ride roller coasters, ride motorcycles, rollerblade, skate, or like the Tarahumara, run down a rocky trail while kicking a rock with your toes. Balance is a huge component of what we do as humans. Indigenous tribes like to do games of balance.

Neuroplastic repair may be the result of neural stimulation provided by balance challenges. I have not found research to support this. I am not a qualified researcher myself. These are just the results I have seen.

If I get a concussion, I have damage to a certain area of my brain. This damage affects the multimodal balance system and all of the intricate communication that goes on in achieving and maintaining balance. So, that damage effectively results in a degradation in balance. To fix the damage, I work in reverse, by fixing my balance. The brain will repair itself as a result.

CONCUSSION PREVENTION

Let's say a young ski racer post-concussion comes to see me. It is his second one in ten months. He scores a 55 on the KBI. It's a good score, but this kid is a hotshot racer. And while his father may think that his balance was fine—his physical therapist had cleared him to ski again, after all—he was well short of the 75 or so that is required to race at the level he does. I believe that he had the second concussion because his body thinks he is still around 75, but it really isn't.

Now, maybe ninety-nine times out of a hundred, he recovers his balance during a race or practice. That's great, but that one time he does fall and lands wrong is all it takes to do severe damage to his brain. And that one time is more likely to happen if his balance level is not where he believes it to be—he no longer has the body awareness to change his position in midfall and mitigate his impact.

If you are engaged in an activity that has large balance demands, perhaps above a 75-point level, and you are operating at a 45–65, you might get away with the first fifty falls or so, but it only takes one bad fall to begin the cycle of concussions. To prevent concussions in higher-risk activities, you must have your balance system appropriately tuned in order to help protect you. I can't prove it, but I believe the first objective of the body in a fall is to protect the head. When one considers the fact that the number-one cause of TBIs is falls, then it is clear that better balance will reduce the number of concussions.

Part Four

THE TRAINING
SYSTEM

CHAPTER 17

The Rules to Effective Balance Training

SAFETY

Always be aware of your surroundings and the potential danger if you have to make a sudden movement or a stumble. Keep the floor clear of things you could trip over. Do all balance training away from any weight equipment. Weight machines are big pieces of iron with prominent edges that will cause injury if you stumble off your balance challenge and hit your head.

WHOLE-BODY MOVEMENT

Good balance involves the whole body. Even as a person stands around doing nothing, muscles from the back of the neck to his or her toes—more than seven hundred of them—are engaged in maintaining balance. So when a person balance-trains, it is important to use the arms and let the body move freely.

I instruct athletes to engage the whole body when working on improving balance. It might look uncoordinated, but this is simply your body finding the right neural firing pattern for better balance. Those big movements will become quiet and more graceful as the neural software organizes a more efficient pattern. So let the arms flail all about.

ATHLETIC POSITION

Nearly all athletic balancing occurs on the front inside third of the foot, with the knee aligned slightly inside the big toe, knees slightly bent, butt sticking out slightly as the body is bent at the hips—not the waist—chest up with shoulders and knees aligned, and feet parallel pointing forward. Never have the toes pointed out.

Having the knee aligned slightly inside the big toe is considered heresy in the fitness world. In all movements involving cutting, turning, striking, and landing, the knee will find its way aligned just inside the big toe. I have looked at thousands of photos of athletes to see this, but more important for my purposes is that I see it in balance training every day.

It might be considered a weaker position for lifting weights, but this knee aligned inside the big toe happens to be a natural position in all athletic movement, and it does improve balance. I believe an athlete should build strength and balance in positions he or she finds him/herself in his or her sport.

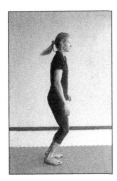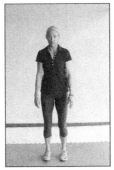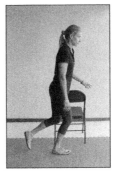

Key point: Never balance on your heels when doing single-foot balancing. Coaches like to cue athletes to put their weight on their heels before certain lifts, but this is exactly the wrong thing to do when working on balance. Remember, nothing athletic ever happens on your heels. There is a phrase in the world of boxing of "having the other guy on his heels." It means the opponent is off-balance.

Try these heel-balance positions shown below. Now try to jump. Try to move off your heels and land on your heels. Now try to jump rope on your heels. Hard, huh? When you are done laughing, return to the athletic position and then try to jump.

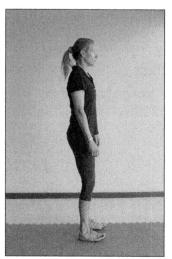 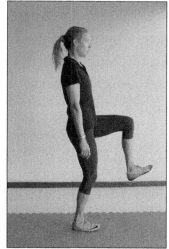

VISION

I have talked about peripheral vision and balance throughout this book, and here it is again. I can demonstrate to my clients, and they immediately understand, that staring at a particular spot works against the sense of balance. Utilize broad vision as if you are looking at a giant painting. If you wear bifocals or progressive glasses, try training without them, and use instead your single-vision glasses or contacts.

When clients begin a new balance challenge, their instinct is to look down. I am fine with that as long as they are utilizing their broad vision. As people get better at it, I will have them raise their heads and look at the horizon while keeping a broad focus, sensing what is at their feet.

WEIGHTS

Weights are not a part of our balance work. This is my direct message: Never lift weights while balance training. When lifting weights, you are preventing the part of the body doing the lifting from engaging in the process of balance, and that's counterproductive. Remember, proper balance training engages the whole body.

Another reason we avoid weights is that most weight-lifting involves bilateral movements utilizing both arms and hands simultaneously. All balance and, in fact, all athletic movements use contralateral movement. Lifting weights while balance training inhibits that contralateral movement.

Finally, lifting weights while attempting to balance is just plain dangerous because effective training of the balance system requires working to the point of falling. You don't want to be on the verge of falling while holding weights, which could fall on you.

CLEAR MIND, NO JUDGMENT, NO MUSIC

Balance comes from the subconscious, non-thinking part of the mind. I may sound like Yoda, but there is no thinking in balance training, no conscious effort, no rah-rah exhorting to do better, and no judgment of performance.

I do not allow music in the gym nor do I allow clients to play music while training. Listening to music artificially shuts off the conscious mind.

One important outcome of training in balance is that it improves your athletic focus, and it allows the intelligence of the body to find the right position on its own. So when my clients start to analyze themselves, I remind them to stop thinking about it.

CHAPTER 18

The Equipment

SAFETY REVIEW

Before you step on a piece of balance equipment with the intent of becoming off-balance, it's important to review the rules of safety.

1. Respect your fear and sense of discomfort. These are not walls to be beaten down, but instead, they signal information about where a client's ability currently stands. The idea of pushing through fear is a popular one. However, fear is an evolutionary trait that was developed for a good reason. So if we see that a client who is preparing to attempt a certain exercise has a high level of fear or discomfort, that usually means the person's body is not ready to perform the feat.

2. Proper balance training is a progression from less difficult to more difficult. Attempting to skip a level is to deny the body an opportunity to learn.

3. Replicate the training facility as closely as possible when doing exercises at home. Have a bar, chair, or wall that you can reach out to to catch your balance. Or have someone spot you. A dining room chair can substitute for a person if you don't have somebody around.

4. Clear the area where you are working. Aside from a dining room chair or spotter, make sure you don't any obstructions on the ground that could be tripped over or that could hurt you if you fell on them. If you're working in a gym, for example, a stack of forty-five-pound barbell plates is a disaster waiting to happen.

5. Turn off the music. Settle into a Zen-like state when you are working on your balance. Save the music for a cycling class or aerobics.

BALANCE-TRAINING EQUIPMENT

Slacklines or SlackBow: You have probably seen a slackline in a photograph or seen someone using it at a campground. A slackline is tied between two objects and is used to balance on. I designed the SlackBow in order to do the same type of balance work in the gym.

With the SlackBow, there are three different heights that

can be used and an infinite number of adjustments that can be made to the tension. Basically, the tighter the line, the more board like, thus reducing movement, which is better for the beginner. The looser and longer the line, the more oscillation, thus making it more difficult.

SlackPlate: For those who have advanced in their balance training, the SlackPlate is a three and half inch wide plate that can be used on top of the SlackBow line to increase the difficulty.

Soft Plyo Box: At gyms, you will see all sorts of plyo boxes, usually the wooden kind. In balance training, we use a soft version of a plyo box. We use them to hop, as if they were rocks on a river. We have exercises that involve moving up and down across the boxes. The softness of the box adds a degree of instability to fire up the balance senses. And because losing balance is part of our protocol, the soft boxes are safer and less threatening to our athletes.

BOSU: A BOSU looks like half of an inflated ball mounted to a large disc. We use the BOSU for two-foot balance with the round side down and the flat side up.

SlackBoards or Balance Boards: This is a balance-training device that uses a board on top of a roller. The athlete stands on the board and performs drills to work on balance skills.

Touch Support: This is simply a chair with a back, wall, barre or even a partner. This can be used as a support in the early stages of a balance-training regime.

CHAPTER 19

Skills Assessment

———

Enough about the theories of why you need better balance. Let's get started. This a three-level plan. This plan should be enough to safely improve your balance to the point where you will notice a difference in your life and the sports you play.

EVALUATING BALANCE

We start balance training with an initial assessment. Before discussing how to do that on your own, let's review the safety precautions, which should be foremost in any program.

Quick note: I've put together a series of videos to support all of the instructions and photos in this book. Log on to www.slackbow.com/readers for information and videos you can work with.

PROGRESSIONS AND SAFETY

There are several key components to balance training. First, balance exercises have to be difficult enough to present a challenge. You need to energize the latent modalities within your sense of balance. If the balance exercises are too mild, you won't get much, if anything, in return.

An example I used previously is that the suggestion that if you lift five pounds a day for a set of twenty, you would get stronger. You just wouldn't get much stronger. The way you get stronger is by increasing weight and repetitions. The same thinking is true in balance training. The balance system improves only if it is properly challenged incrementally as one's ability progresses.

What does this have to do with safety? A true progressive balance-challenge will take you to a point of failure. In terms of human balance, failure means a fall or a near-fall. What is unique about the SlackBow Balance Training methods, however, is that these protocols will take a person to the point of failure without falling or having a near-fall. Please note, however, that if you decide to jump ahead on the progression scale, you are risking a fall.

Start with the evaluation, then progress through the levels even if you think you can go ahead and move on to level 2 or 3.

Always train in an area that is clear of obstacles. Clear the floor of things you could trip on, such as a stray kettlebell or medicine ball. Even though we never have falls at our facility, we still keep a safe space just in case there is one. During SlackBow Balance Training, we are always scanning the floor and the area to be sure that if a client has to step off or does fall, the area is clear.

I see people in gyms balance training right next to weight machines with heavy steel and sharp edges. I know of a famous skier who used to balance-train near heavy equipment. Well, she went down one day and had to get stitches on her pretty face. When balance training, always be scanning for what might happen if you do lose your balance. Either move it out of the way or move yourself to a different area.

We prefer our clients to wear minimalist athletic shoes with the thinnest soles possible and a zero-heel drop. Most clients do not have this type of athletic shoe, so we then require they train barefoot. The safety issue here is to never train with just socks, as they are way too slippery to train in.

When beginning a new balance challenge, always have a safety support nearby. That safety support can be a wall, chair, barre bar, or training buddy who you can reach out and touch. You don't want to lean on these, but you do want them close enough to reach out and touch for support if necessary. Never train without a safety support.

BALANCE TRAINING: ARE YOU A CANDIDATE?

The purpose of the evaluation is to discover if you are ready to begin the SlackBow Balance Training program. This is not the classic medical balance evaluation. If you are having serious balance issues, I recommend you seek the guidance of a physical therapist or doctor.

The first step in the evaluation is to answer the following yes-or-no questions.

1. Are you under a doctor's care for lower extremity injury or a medical condition that affects your balance?
2. Are you working with a physical therapist, actively rehabbing an injury from an accident or surgery?
3. Do you need to use a walker, cane, crutches, walking stick, or some sort of aid to help when you walk?
4. Do you shuffle your feet when you walk?
5. Are you over forty-five and with an injury-causing fall in the last six months?

If you answered yes to any of these questions, I suggest you not begin this program now. If you are under a doctor's care, ask if it is OK to begin this balance program. If you are working with a physical therapist, wait until you have finished your physical therapy to begin balance training.

Physical therapists often incorporate balance training in their protocols, but the SlackBow program involves more-demanding balance challenges and is designed to deliver results for athletes. It is best to start after you have completed all your physical therapy sessions and get the go-ahead from your physical therapist.

I work with clients who need some sort of aid when walking, but it is a very different training and not something I would recommend you try after simply reading my book. Working with a balance-qualified physical therapist would be a good place to start.

If you are over forty-five and have had an injury-causing fall in the last six months, I would consider you at risk with your balance system. You can proceed with the program, but exercise caution.

Below is the evaluation. For more details and support videos, please refer to SlackBow.com/reader.

EVALUATION

Be sure to have the proper safety setup like the ones in the photos below.

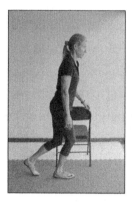 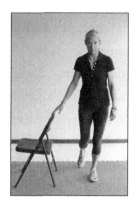

Begin by getting into the athletic position. The athletic position includes the following body positions:

- Weight forward on the inside front of your feet
- Knees slightly bent
- Bend at the hips, not the waist; stick your butt out slightly
- Chest up

Here is an easy way to get into that position; do the following without any forethought or plan. In other words, perform them as naturally as you can. Hop slightly off the ground three times. After the third time, land and just hold that position. That is your athletic position. Refer to video at slackbow.com

Now that you are in the athletic position, hold on to your safety support, then take your left leg and move it backward to where your left big toe is a few inches behind the right heel. Lift your left foot slightly off the ground, maybe three inches, and balance on your front foot. Take your hand off your support, and see how long you can stay in that position.

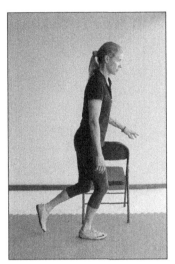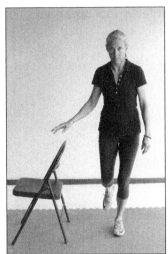

Do the same with the other foot.

TEST

Stay on one foot for fifteen seconds without the other foot touching the floor or your hand touching the support.

When you can do this on each foot, then you are ready to do level 1.

For those of you who think, "I am really good. I'll just jump to level 3," please humor me, and quickly and competently buzz through levels 1 and 2. Then do level 3 if you wish. The progression is essential to safety and is the best way to improve your balance. Being patient and methodical will pay the most dividends in your balance training.

CHAPTER 20

Level 1 Balance Training

Time to get started. For the first level of the SlackBow Balance Training program, you won't need much in the way of equipment. But let's review the best practices to get the most out of your training investment.

This is simply a strong start to a lifetime of balance training. Mastering the three-level program laid out in this book will give you a reboot of your inner balance operating system and provide you with the tools and understanding to make improvements on your own.

So you've performed the evaluation, and you're ready to begin level 1. Even if you are a balance hotshot, I strongly advise working through each phase of the three-level program.

We start with a basic eight-minute routine. In the first level of training, we will do exercises called "side to sides" and "step-throughs."

THE EIGHT-MINUTE ROUTINE

EQUIPMENT:

This exercise is done on the floor with your safety touch support, such as a dining room chair. Set an interval timer for two minutes.

EXERCISE:

This may seem easy, but I promise it is harder than you imagine. Just like in the test, get into the athletic position. Next, move your left foot back to where your left toe is aligned with your right heel. With your support nearby, lift your left foot just a few inches off the ground, and balance on the right foot as long as you can. If your foot touches or you touch the support, just start again. You are not trying to set a record or go the full two minutes. Keep doing these attempts for two minutes on each side.

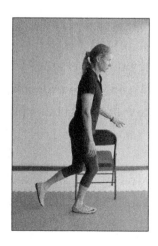

FRONT AND BACK BALANCE

EQUIPMENT:
Chair back

EXERCISE:
This exercise is similar, but you won't be in the athletic position. You will be in what I call the "fall" position. Sounds scary, right? Don't worry, it's not.

Place your chair or support about two to three feet in front of you.

Start in the athletic position. Next, take the left foot and move it so that your left big toe is two foot-lengths aligned behind your right heel. This will force you to bend at the waist and actually look at the ground. This is the only exercise in which you will bend at the waist and look at the ground. The objective is to use the front part of your foot for balance.

Next, reach out with your hands and touch your support. At the same time, lift your foot a couple of inches off the ground and lift your hand off the support. Hold for as long as you can. Repeat attempts for two minutes, then do it with the other leg.

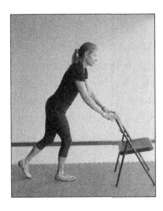 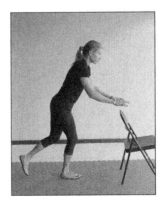

SIDE TO SIDES

EQUIPMENT:
Floor

EXERCISE:
Stand with feet shoulder-width apart in the athletic position.

Gently leap to a point six inches out from your left foot, hold the position on one left foot for a second, then leap to the same distance in out from your right foot and hold on the right foot for one second. Repeat twenty times in a slow, controlled manner. Every time you land, drop down more in your athletic position to absorb the energy of the landing. Land on the inside front-third of your foot.

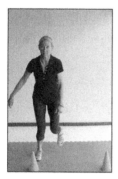 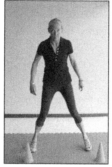 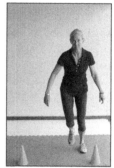

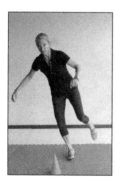

If you are landing and rolling to the outside of your foot, you are out of balance. Once you are on the outside edge of your foot, you are no longer in balance. It is similar to being on your heels. If you are doing this (see photo), shorten your leap distance or drop down more to absorb the landing energy and consciously work to land on the inside of the foot lined up just inside the knee.

STEP-THROUGHS

EQUIPMENT:

One or two bath towels folded into quarters, about four inches in height or a foam pad like the one in the photos. Set your support nearby. Set the towel to your right side, in line where you will step on it with your right foot.

EXERCISE:

Take a step with your right foot and land on the towel in an athletic position on the front part of your foot. Try to land on your forefoot. Hold in that position on the towel for one second. Step on the towel; say, "one, one thousand"; and then step off the towel and onto your left foot.

Turn around and do the same with your left foot. Do this for two minutes or until tired.

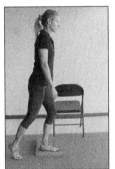 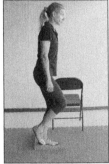 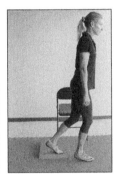

CHAPTER 21

Level 2 Balance Training

Once you can perform the level 1 exercises well and for the designated amounts of time, it is time to progress to level 2. You will start again with the same eight-minute routine that you did at level 1 but with a little kick to it.

EIGHT-MINUTE ROUTINE PLUS

This is the same routine from level 1 introduced in the previous chapter, but you will perform the routine by upping the ante—and the challenge—by performing the exercises on an unstable platform. Take a look at the videos at slackbow.com/reader for additional instruction.

EQUIPMENT OPTIONS:

Safety support, stack of folded bath towels no higher than six inches.

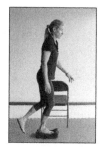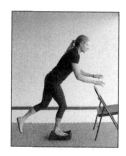

Airex pad (a thick foam pad designed for balance training—easy to find on Amazon) or similar thick foam pad.

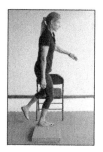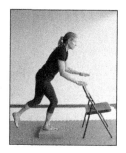

SlackBlock (you can find the SlackBlock on my website at slackbow.com)

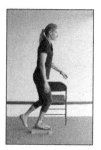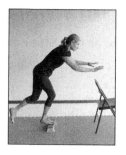

Select either the folded towel, the Airex pad, or the SlackBlock, along with your safety support, and do the eight-minute routine. Have your support nearby when starting with this exercise. The idea is to stimulate your sense of balance back to life through neurological confusion; to do this, you must edge toward a state of losing your balance.

SIDE TO SIDES

EQUIPMENT:
Floor

EXERCISE:
Side to sides as before, but work to stretch out the distance in your leaps. Always remain in control by absorbing the landing and staying on the inside of your foot. Do this for two minutes.

FRONT TO FRONT

Leap from your right foot forward this time onto your left. Absorb the landing by dropping into the athletic position. Hold it for a count of one, then leap onto your right and continue for twenty on each side.

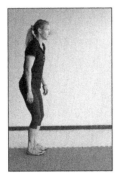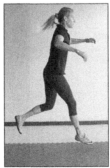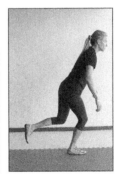

In both of these exercises, maintain your athletic position—bent knees, springy crouch, head up, on the balls of your feet.

MULTISENSE NEURAL LOADING

EQUIPMENT:

Same equipment as in level 2
Tennis ball, basketball (any ball that can be bounced), or tossing beanbag

EXERCISE:

There's a prerequisite for Multisense Neural Loading: Only do this exercise if you can execute the level 2 eight-minute routine without safety support.

Stand on your chosen unstable platform on one foot. While in this position, bounce pass the tennis ball against the wall and catch it when it comes back. Or bounce a basketball or any ball on the ground and catch it. If you have a partner, play catch with the beanbag. Do this for two minutes on each foot.

The key to this exercise is to use broad vision and see the ball in the big picture you are looking at.

In time, you will be catching the ball without directly looking at it. My young clients call it "zombie eyes."

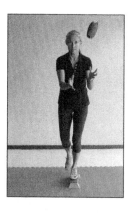 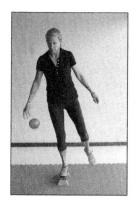

CHAPTER 22

Level 3 Balance Training

———

Level 3 is a big jump. The equipment is going to make the challenges much more difficult. More than anything, I want you to be fully comfortable in your level 2 skills and be sure to follow the safety protocol on all level 3 exercises.

FOUR-MINUTE ROUTINE

EQUIPMENT:
Aerobics step box

SAFETY SUPPORT:
A slackline or SlackBow

Slackline: The slackline setup should be a two-inch line stretched as tight as possible with a length between twelve and sixteen feet long. The height of the line above the ground should be no higher than twelve to fifteen inches. Place the aerobic step box next to the line. Place the safety support on the other side.

When setting up the slackline, put a square of carpet or rug in between the tree and the line to protect the bark of the tree.

There are some great slackline companies, a list of whose products can be found at slackbow.com

SlackBow: This piece of equipment is something I developed with six college seniors majoring in engineering. The SlackBow is a patented slackline frame that comes in two lengths: 12.5 feet and 15 feet. It has three height adjustments and is infinitely adjustable from very tight to very loose, which is to say, easier to harder. It can hold more than six hundred pounds. In fact, I have had two 300-pound-plus football linemen on it at the same time. Go to slackbow.com for more information.

Set the SlackBow at the lowest height with the line as tight as possible. Place the aerobic step box on one side and the safety support on the other side.

EXERCISES:
The left-to-right-to-left, side-to-side balance position is called the "parallel position" on the line. With the right foot on the line, the big toe of the left foot is lined up on the box behind the right heel.

To begin, lift your left foot off the box an inch or two, then touch back down. Keep your hand on the safety support.

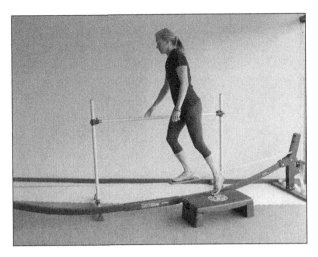

Next, lift your hand off the safety support, then lift your left foot off the box. Keep doing this until you feel comfortable enough to move the safety support out of the way. I have never had a client fall off the SlackBow. Don't worry about falling. If you have done your progression to this point, you will find that your body has a very good messaging system, which will alert you that you have lost your balance, allowing you to step off long before you would fall.

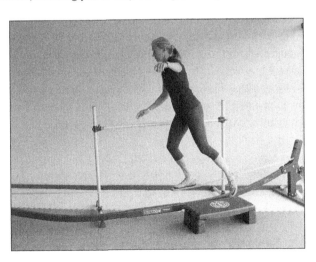

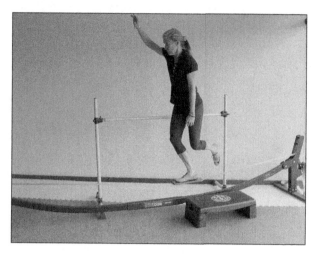

The whole body needs to be free to move. The bigger the motion, the faster you will improve your balance. Do not try to control any motion. Let the body's intelligence do its job.

BALANCE BOARDS

EQUIPMENT:

There are many companies that sell great balance boards. They are all offshoots of the original Bongo Board. I first started on a Bongo Board in 1960. As a child with severe attention deficit disorder, my dad would challenge me to see how long I could stay up on the board. All balance board brands have their own unique benefits. I tried them all and found that they are each good for their own purpose, but for my protocols and balance-training athletes of all ages in a gym environment, I designed a board that would satisfy all of my needs.

Balance boards are dangerous without proper training. I would not feel comfortable teaching you how to use it merely by writing about it. Instead, I want you to learn by watching. Get your balance board and go to slackbow.com for an instructional video.

Code to access the book videos is "BIP" in caps.

CONCLUSION

A Balanced Life

It seems strange that our balance system, that uniquely human attribute, remains so hidden and unexamined. What we are capable of doing on two feet and even on one foot, what we do in sports and in our daily lives is nothing short of amazing.

Balance occupies a staggering percentage of our overall neural system. And it is the neural system, rather than just the brain or the body, as a whole. In practice, there is a brain in the lower back, a brain in the stomach, and so on. When integrated and in sync in a natural, outdoor environment, we feel better. This is why when we sit in our chairs in our offices under our fluorescent lighting, we wish that we are outside.

And that is central to the final message I want to impart

about training: be an athlete all the time.

I find it ironic when I see athletes go practice a sport or do a workout, and then leave the gym and move like someone who has never participated in athletics. Why not walk athletically and incorporate athletic activities into your everyday life?

When you're on a train, can you stand still and not hold on to the post? When you're on a boat, can you stand with your knees bent, balancing as the waves rock the boat? Can you move fluidly through different spaces on different terrains? We can apply the basics of balance training all the time in our daily lives.

Use an athletic stance.

Look up.

Use broad vision.

Be loose; relax away tensions and use a springy style of movement.

Once you integrate these principles into everything you do, you can, for example, get up from your desk, step back and look at your computer, and do a spot check: I've got my broad vision, I can see everything, I'm on my toes, I'm balancing on one foot, and my mind goes quiet.

To take it up a level, stash a folded towel in your office desk or a SlackBlock underneath it and make it part of your ritual. Maybe you're just doing this for a second or two every hour or so, but this is all it takes to fire up your balance system. And to polish it all off, have a plant on your desk to break up the weariness of the typical—and deadening—geometry of the workplace.

The following are some things to do and one thing to not do.

My one "don't" is one that I've heard recommended time and time again to improve balance, and it's putting your socks and shoes on while standing. This is not a good balance-training activity. I used to do it and always hated it because I was not very good at it. And I am sure there are few people in the world at my age, if any, with my balance skills.

Then it dawned on me: When doing this, you are in the most unnatural and worst balance position possible. You are on your heel on one leg, with the other leg bent in front of you while you are completely bending at the waist. Then to top that off, you are doing it in a bedroom or dressing room with all sorts of bad things to fall on and hurt yourself. Oh, and yeah, when you are putting on your shoes, you are in your slippery socks. Brilliant—NOT. Don't do this.

So, here are some things you can do:

Stand up every now and then. Stand on one foot, then the other, maintaining the athletic position. Allow your body to be loose and relaxed. You'll be surprised at how this clears your mind.

If you are standing around, feel where the pressure is on your feet. If you feel all the pressure on your heels, then you are not in a good balance position. Try to stand in the athletic position with the weight on the forward part of your feet.

When riding up (not down) an escalator, stand on one foot in the athletic position. Don't hold the handrail, but hover your hand above it for safety. You will be shocked at how difficult this it.

Walk down stairs with your eyes up. To be safe, look down first and always look down if you have an instinct to do so; but after you look down, look up again to engage your peripheral vision as you walk down the stairs. Don't hold the railing, but please be sure to hover your hand above the railing for safety. Do not do this if you wear progressive or bifocal glasses.

Ride airport terminal trams and trains without holding on to a support. Be in the athletic position with your weight on the inside forward part of your feet. Do this with both feet on the ground. Be near a pole that you can reach out to to catch yourself if you do lose your balance.

You will begin to find your own daily balance activities. And I'd love to hear about it. Please visit my blog, and let me know what you've thought up and how your overall balance-training program is going. Visit me at slackbow.com

The SlackBow Balance Training System

I have always considered myself to be a giant klutz with very poor balance. I thought that good balance was something that you had to be born with and could not learn.

I met Jim when he ordered some coats from my company. I went to his balance studio to meet him and discuss the job and he showed me around. I was instantly intrigued. In Park city we have every work out, fitness, diet and exercise program imaginable, but no one had focused only on balance. I had to try it and was astounded with the results.

The workouts were really fun, incredibly challenging, and

vigorous. After an hour session my limbs were shaking, I was sweating, but my heart was elated. Each time I was pushed well out of my comfort zone, but NEVER felt endangered. Jim or Janet were there by my side, always ready to spot or catch me, and were masters at getting me to believe in myself enough that I could push to the next level. I felt that my improvement was astounding. And even though I had long periods of time between each session I felt like I never backslid, and I could take up each time where I left off.

The most amazing thing for me was the crossover effect it had on other sports in my life. I am a passionate skier. I love any type of skiing: powder, moguls, steeps and cliffs, and especially ski racing slalom and GS. The first day on snow after my fall SlackBow sessions was unreal. I felt like I was on a new improved set of legs. I have been skiing since age 2 and have always felt comfortable on skis. But now I felt rock solid. Everything just seemed easier. Flat light was not as difficult. Committing to the fall line, pressuring the outside ski, moving into the next turn, going over rough terrain or icy slopes and bumps was just easier. I was skiing with a new level of confidence. I now feel like I no longer look at each part of the slope thinking here is a bump, watch the compression, its icy here etc but rather just dance over the terrain. Probably the best tell was my husband. He has been a ski racing coach for 30 years, coaching everything from little kids to US ski team. He does not give praise easily. After watching me ski one day that winter he shook his head and said, "what happened to you? You are skiing like one of my FIS kids"—this is an unimaginably HUGE compliment from a crusty German Schilehrer—I just smiled and said "SLACKBOW."

This summer we went to Alaska and backpacked the Chilkoot trail. This is not a hike for the faint of heart. We had a lot of rain. So the streams we had to cross were deep rushing cold torrents. We had to jump from boulder to boulder carrying a 45 pound backpack and a misstep or slip and fall could have been disastrous or even fatal. We also hiked through miles of steep slippery wet boulder fields and snowfields that were converted to glare ice because of the rain. When we hit the streams I channeled Jim's Rover Rocks training took a deep breath and hopped across. My new improved ski legs got me through the snow fields, and the confidence I gained on the SlackBow and SlackBoard got me over all of those slippery boulder fields, and this was after I watched a hiker in front of me slip and fall and break her leg.

Finally, I am an Emergency Physician who has worked in emergency rooms for over 25 years. Falls, especially among the elderly, are a major cause of morbidity and mortality in our country. The cost of injuries secondary to falls whether it is the actual medical bill, cost of lost productivity, or cost to care for people who are no longer able to live in their homes because of disability secondary to the fall is astronomical. One also has to consider the emotional cost to patients and their families when they can no longer be self-sufficient. While balance training is great for athletes, If I was queen of the world, I would make it a mandatory part of our health care system for anyone over the age of 55. I am a strong believer that the long term physical improvement that we would see in a elderly population who has had good balance and strength training would greatly offset any cost that program might incur.

— CELESTE RAFFIN, MD

Your SlackBow Balancing System has revolutionized my approach to Balance Training. The SlackBow system focuses on the ability of the brain to find the correct balance position for each new activity. As a result, I have developed a more intuitive, proprioceptive response to off-balance body positions.

— RANDY

The first time I tried to balance on the SlackBow, the line was relatively tight, and by applying most of my weight to the foot of my right leg that is placed on the line, my leg began to shake substantially in the side-to-side direction. There was no way I was going to stand or attempt to balance on the line for more than a second. I had little to no balance. I literally looked like Charles Barkley trying to hit a golf ball. As a matter of fact, I grew up playing golf with my grandfather and played in high school. I certainly was not the best; however, I knew how to swing a golf club correctly, etc.

So, when Jim mentioned that I would see positive results when it came to golf, I was definitely determined to learn and train myself in order to have much better balance. Indeed, I was aware of the other balancing tools on the market (and could generally balance on them), but I was less interested in them since it was very easy to achieve and the results were slim. Obviously, I had some work to do to have the capability to balance on the SlackBow for more than a second.

After training on the line for a few sessions, I could already see results. I was walking differently. Not on the balls of my feet, more on the front portions. My posture seemed to be better. I felt more grounded to the floor, feeling more confident when I was walking, turning, or doing anything else on my feet. My legs were stronger and my joints weren't tight. I truly felt better overall, and most definitely regarding my balance. I could also see positive results in my golf game. Since I was more grounded and my balance was much better, I could remain calm while I swung, generally producing a much more fluid swing and an overall more accurate shot. I also saw results with my putting game. The feeling of being grounded after being on the SlackBow is hard to compare with anything else I've ever done in life. I definitely recommend it for anyone seeking that feeling of being grounded, better balance and strength, or for the challenge.

— BLAKE

Quite a few years after my career as a professional ballet dancer and a few after a shorter stint as a Certified Personal Trainer, I thought I knew a thing or two about balance from my training in these two areas. Especially when I began training older adults, including yours truly. I observed first-hand how older people (me included) struggled with balance, sometimes with serious injuries. With younger ballet dancers, you are constantly challenging your balance with an endless variety of movement.

Back to us older folks. I cannot underestimate the importance of good balance as to the quality and safety of your life. Jim Klopman, through his research and innovative thinking in and out of the box, has brought this critical life issue into a broader and more complete understanding. One that people can understand and prevent falls that can change a life significantly. Jim's knowledge and training methods, I believe, reach far beyond conventional and traditional thinking. I hope you have the opportunity to learn from Jim Klopman. He will keep you on your dancing feet! This extraordinary man is for real.

— FRED SCHWAB (84 YEARS AND
STILL MOVIN' ALONG)

At the ripe young age of 69, I am acutely aware of the importance of balance, not only in everyday life situations but also in recreation activities. I also believe that you can "practice" balance exercises designed to improve your instinctive reactions in this area.

The SlackBow approach does just that. And as an extra bonus, the SlackBow improves your performance in recreation activities, from golfing, skiing, and hiking.

— TOM

I believe the statistics are that one out of three people over 65 fall each year. Keeping active requires balance. I am 72 years old (physically, but I still feel like I am 21). I want to stay active. I ski full time in the winter and do other outdoor activities and exercise classes in the summer. I attended a number of SlackBow classes in Park City with Jim as the adviser/teacher. In standing on the SlackBow on one foot, I went from raising my other foot for a millisecond to doing it for single digits of seconds. That is a huge improvement. I skied faster without consciously trying to. Jim's advice on posture and focus was invaluable. Using the SlackBow to teach the balance sensors— ears, vision, and proprioceptors—to fire the small muscles and reduce the shaking that happens due to repetition—not cognitive thinking. Balance can be improved with training. Jim knows the tools to train with.

— CALVIN

I suffered from gout for 20 years, and it caused extensive damage to the joints in my toes, ankles, and knees. When I finally started taking medicine for it, the pain subsided, but I discovered I still had significant postural alignment and balance issues. SlackBow Balance Training was an essential part of my rehabilitation, allowing me to regain a normal gait and much of my flexibility. Now, not only can I hike mountains to my heart's content, I'm able to ski as hard and fast as I want, and my golf game is improved, even down to my putting.

— JEFF

I started SlackBow Training a year after sustaining a concussion. I hate to preach, but in terms of active recovery, it set me further ahead than any other therapy I went through to get me back to daily life.

I had been an NCAA athlete, but my recovery from the concussion had failed to be properly overseen by trainers, and I was still struggling with daily tasks. I began seeking help from outlets ranging from vision therapy to multiple neural specialists.

At the end of the day, SlackBow was the best active treatment I found both cognitively and physically—both elements of my health that were extremely damaged.

As an athlete, having an obtainable goal of an hour of Slack-Bow Training which was healthy and also showing rapid progress toward my health when all other outlets were causing pain and fatigue was hugely successful toward my recovery.

I cannot speak for the science, only my experience. After a year of struggling to function on a day-to-day basis, Slack-Bow started providing a turning point by bringing back my coordination, balance, focus, attention span, and ability to process the environment around me—all things people with functioning brains think are very simple tasks!

SlackBow was providing stimulation for my body and brain. Balance causes every muscle in your body to fire, as you are never in balance but constantly readjusting to stay balanced. These processes fire your mind and your body in a natural, subtle, healthy environment.

On the days I was unsure I was going to be able to get out of bed due to pain, I made it my goal to SlackBow for 10 minutes. That 10 minutes would bring my alertness to a new level that no other activity could by firing my muscles and my brain. Therefore, SlackBow would give me my greatest chance at a successful day. Other sports or activities, even on low levels, required elevated heart rates that caused headaches, speed that caused vision pain, or my other option was no movement, causing stagnant progress. SlackBow provided a solution to all of these things—helped to retrain my vision and focus, a controlled heart rate, no danger of further injury, while also working to fix my vertigo.

My first SlackBow session was a year ago. I am still working through postconcussion symptoms, and in a perfect world, I would be able to SlackBow daily. While I travel, I am attempting to incorporate what I have learned into my daily schedule. I incorporate all of my new knowledge into my coaching techniques, and as an athlete, I wish I had known what I know now at 15. I think it would have positively impacted my entire athletic career.

I have nothing but positive things to say about SlackBow as someone working through long-term concussion symptoms, an athlete, and as a coach. I wish I had been introduced to SlackBow years earlier.

— TAYLOR

I am so glad I met Jim Klopman and was introduced to his product, the SlackBow. As an athlete, I am always looking for ways to differentiate myself from other athletes. Like so many others, I was lifting a lot of weight and getting stronger and found that with greater balance comes greater strength. Lack of balance discounts your potential strength. My time on the SlackBow served me well in more than just my primary sports.

Other than my dedication to baseball, my ability to surf and ski have benefited from this unique training. Something so simple provides such an intense workout in a short amount of time. Simple doesn't mean easy; put some focus and effort into the SlackBow, and you will see the results. When I started training with Jim, he measured my vertical and promised an improvement of a few inches. Sure enough, a couple months later I had recorded a jump 4 inches higher than my best jump prior to SlackBow training. This unique method of training gives you that edge over your opponents. Balancing on the SlackBow fires your fast twitch muscles and really puts entire body and mind to work.

— CHANDLER

I have been skiing for over 50 years, 40 of them at PCMR. For the last 20 years I have been a part of a gang that skies every Tuesday morning before we go to Rotary lunch. I am an expert skier, but after passing age 60, I noticed that I was slowing down; over the years with the same gang, I was slowly moving further back in the pack on arrival at the lift. Part of this was that some younger folks had joined in over the years.

Jim did a demo of SlackBow for our Rotary club and then invited us in for a private session. I had a one-hour visit where Jim put me through the entire spectrum of activities he had devised. The following week, skiing with the same bunch in same conditions, I found myself standing at the lift at the bottom of the hill waiting for the gang to catch up. One of the gang is the father of the world champion ski racer and a very fine skier—my age—himself.

I never would have believed that this simple training could produce such outstanding results.

— KEVIN

I don't have any data to back this up—no controlled tests to validate improvement over time. All I can say is that using the SlackBow to improve my balance has contributed to a heightened mental state that when engaged in active sports, has had a positive impact on my performance and my mental attitude. Yes, I feel (physically) stronger. Yes, I feel more in (psychological) control. Yes, I am more confident when I:

Swing a golf club.
Transfer weight from ski to ski.
Control my bike on a technical downhill ride.
Need the inner peace required to navigate personal relationships.

To me, it's the most efficient workout—both physically and mentally.

— JOE

Working with Jim has changed the way I do many everyday things. I walk as an athlete—no more laid-back heel striking. I ski with better balance, and I'm more aware of my posture. I even observe bad posture and sometimes get upset! Jim understands the body and what it takes to keep the body lasting and performing at a high level. He also makes it fun.

— ED

My name is Jim Black, and I was a professional ski instructor for 24 years, first in New England, then in Utah. As I have gotten older, my skill level has diminished, so I decided to take one of Jim Klopman's SlackBow courses, and it was everything I hoped it would be. I felt much more comfortable on my skis, especially at speed or in difficult conditions, and overall much more balanced and sure of myself. I found it also helped my cycling, both road and mountain.

I may not be 25 anymore, but I am skiing better than I have in years.

— JIM BLACK

I was in Machu Picchu and was climbing the tall mountain that everyone sees in the pictures. The trail was incredibly steep and rocky. Everyone I was with felt shaky on these steep trails. Normally, I would have felt the same. Lucky for me, I had been using the SlackBow. My balance was amazing. I was not worried if there was a slight shift in my center of gravity or balance. I knew I could handle it. I simply felt much more confident. Truly stupendous. Thank you so much for this fabulous invention.

— DR. ROBERT SCHWARZ, EXECUTIVE DIRECTOR, ASSOCIATION FOR COMPREHENSIVE ENERGY PSYCHOLOGY

I'm not someone who ever really thought about balance. Mine was pretty good, I thought, owing to good genes from my athletic parents, which I then passed on to my children, two of whom became Division I athletes. So when I happened on Jim's SlackBow studio in Park City, I was intrigued—and totally unprepared for the challenge that followed.

Training with Jim was a physical workout unlike any I had ever experienced. I felt like I was working my muscles hard, but there was never any soreness. I hardly broke a sweat during the workout, but the evening after, I would feel mentally exhausted, go to bed early, and sleep like a baby.

It didn't take long for me to start seeing an impact on my performance in sports I thought I had already mastered. My tennis serve was faster, my return of serve quicker. I could drive a golf ball farther. But most surprising of all was that even five months after I'd completed my series of workouts, I found myself skiing faster, even on the first day of the season.

At first, I thought it was because my ankles felt stronger, but it then dawned on me that I was able to transfer my weight more efficiently from one ski to the other and carve my turns like never before. That's when I remembered: it must have been the balance training that made the difference! That was all the proof I needed. Balance became my religion, and I've been eager ever since to spread the word.

I spent several weeks training with Jim and Janet in Park City over a summer, but went back to New York in September with just a small foam block to practice with. One day, I foolishly climbed up on a high marble window sill in my socks to investigate a leak, and my foot slipped, sending me tumbling backward, head first toward a disastrous impact with the floor. Suddenly, I felt like I was moving in slow motion as I managed to twist myself around, break my fall by stepping on the seat of my desk chair, and hitting the floor on my padded flank.

I thought it was a miracle that instead of breaking my neck, I had nothing more than a nasty black and blue mark on my thigh. Then I realized it was not a miracle but the balance training that had taught me, unconsciously, how to fall without hurting myself.

Even the uneven sidewalks of New York City are no match for me now! I'm convinced more than ever that everyone needs balance training—especially aging baby boomers like me.

— SUSAN

Acknowledgments

===

Thank you to the following individuals; who without their contributions and support, this book would not have been written:

Zach Obront, Tucker Max and the team from Book In A Box. If you have a book in you, this company will make it happen.

Susan Ades Stone for giving so much of her time to make this book happen, even though she would occasionally hurt my feelings.

To Janet, Betsy and Jim Sanders, and Katie and Drew Fike for always being there to help with anything relating to this book and SlackBow.

Thank you to the following individuals; who without their contributions and support, the SlackBow Balance Training System would not have succeeded:

Josh Jones, Hal Richardson and Nancy Klopman for their early support. Rob Engle Ph.D, Stacey Marble, De'varus May, Matt Kirk, Blake Hudson and Chris Kelly for their help in developing the SlackBow. Brian Wright, Ph.D. at Auburn's Office of Technology Transfer Auburn University for his patience and guidance. Pam and Doug Jepperson of Park City Karate. Michael Stephenson for being a great cheerleader and believer. Jake Sweeney of Jake's House of Iron, John Jarman of Summit Strength and Conditioning, Jeff Stone, Ben Herbert NCCA College strength and conditioning coach, Lizzy Galbo, Robert Schwarz, Greg Nicosia, Carole Stern, Brad Stell, Brad Groff, Brad Mooneyham, Lynn Roach, Troy Kelly, Harry Adelson, Dixie Johnson and Marty and Lynn Shattuck. Thanks you to all my clients who each seem to be smarter than the average person.

About the Authors

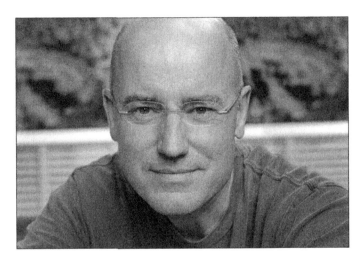

JIM KLOPMAN

Jim Klopman is an innovator who says that his brain damage, ADHD and dyslexia are blessings that free his mind to see tech advances before others. Jim developed the SlackBow Balance Training System to improve and maintain his own athletic performance so he could be athletic all the way into his 90s.

After five years of development, Jim knows that with the right neural whole body training to optimize the human balance system, every person will improve in sport, brain function, longevity, and will feel younger.

Jim puts his own training to use. If you go skiing in Park City where he lives, he will probably fly by you on the slope.

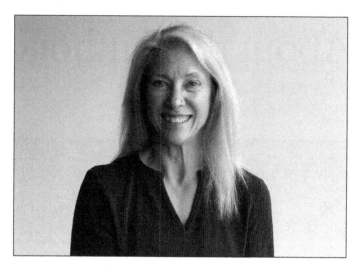

JANET MILLER

Janet Miller is a former body builder who has been a highly innovative personal trainer in hyper fit focused Park City for over 25 years. She was the first to bring spinning to town and has always had an eye for what is best in fitness.

After discovering SlackBow Balance Training, she knew it was the secret all athletic performance. Since adding the training to her clients' routines, she has repeatedly seen amazing outcomes in improving her clients' lives.

Janet puts her training to use as one of Park City's top mountain bikers. If you ride in Park City, she will pass you going up a steep trail. When she does, take a look at her rear wheel, and you may realize that you were passed by rider on a single speed bike!

Made in the USA
Columbia, SC
14 June 2023

18072560R00124